T4-AIL-010

Critical Thinking
in the
Pediatric
Unit

Skills to Assess, Analyze, and Act

Shelley Cohen, RN, BS, CEN

Critical Thinking in the Pediatric Unit: Skills to Assess, Analyze, and Act is published by HCPro, Inc.

Copyright ©2007 HCPro, Inc.

All rights reserved. Printed in the United States of America.   5   4   3   2   1

ISBN: 978-1-57839-952-9

No part of this publication may be reproduced, in any form or by any means, without prior written consent of HCPro, Inc., or the Copyright Clearance Center (978/750-8400). Please notify us immediately if you have received an unauthorized copy.

HCPro, Inc., provides information resources for the healthcare industry.

HCPro, Inc. is not affiliated in any way with The Joint Commission, which owns the JCAHO and Joint Commission trademarks.

Shelley Cohen, RN, BS, CEN, Author
Polly Gerber Zimmermann, RN, MS, MBA, CEN, Contributing Author
June Marshall, RN, MS, CNAA,BC, Contributing Author
Rebecca Hendren, Managing Editor
Emily Sheahan, Group Publisher
Patrick Campagnone, Cover Designer
Paul Singer, Graphic Artist
Mike Mirabello, Senior Graphic Artist
Jean St. Pierre, Director of Operations
Darren Kelly, Production Coordinator

Advice given is general. Readers should consult professional counsel for specific legal, ethical, or clinical questions.

Arrangements can be made for quantity discounts. For more information, contact

HCPro, Inc.
P.O. Box 1168
Marblehead, MA 01945
Telephone: 800/650-6787 or 781/639-1872
Fax: 781/639-2982
E-mail: *customerservice@hcpro.com*

Visit HCPro, Inc., at its World Wide Web sites: *www.hcpro.com* and *www.hcmarketplace.com*

Contents

Contents

Contents

List of figures

Chapter 9

About the authors

Shelley Cohen, RN, BS, CEN

Shelley Cohen, RN, BS, CEN, is the founder and president of Health Resources Unlimited, a Tennessee-based healthcare education and consulting company (*www.hru.net*). Through her seminars for nursing professionals, Cohen coaches and educates healthcare workers and leaders across the country to provide the very best in patient care. She frequently presents her work on leadership and triage at national conferences.

When she is not speaking or teaching, Cohen works as a staff emergency department nurse and develops educational plans for a local emergency department, including strategies for new-graduate orientation. She also writes her monthly electronic publications—*Manager Tip of the Month* and *Triage Tip of the Month*—read by thousands of professionals across the United States.

She is an editorial advisor for *Strategies for Nurse Managers*, published by HCPro, Inc., and is a frequent contributor to *Nursing Management* magazine. She is the author of *Critical Thinking in the Emergency Department* and *Critical Thinking in the Obstetrics Unit*, and co-authored the book *A Practical Guide to Recruitment and Retention: Skills for Nurse Managers*, all published by HCPro, Inc.

She has a background in emergency, critical care, and occupational medicine. Over the past 30 years, she has worked both as a staff nurse and nurse executive.

When her laptop computer shuts down and her stethoscope comes off, Cohen puts on her child-advocacy hat and, with the help of her husband, Dennis, provides foster care to area children.

Contributing author: Polly Gerber Zimmermann, RN, MS, MBA, CEN

Polly Gerber Zimmermann, RN, MS, MBA, CEN, has been in active in emergency and medical-surgical nursing clinical practice for more than 29 years and involved in nurse educating for more than 10 years. She was the senior course manager for the nursing division of the National Center for Advanced Medical Education, and is a tenured assistant professor in the Department of Nursing at the Harry S. Truman College (Chicago). Under her guidance, the school's curriculum instituted an integration of prioritization principles and critical thinking that resulted in the school's students improving from below to above national average results in these areas on standardized test scores.

Zimmermann is a frequent national speaker and has published more than 200 times. In addition, she writes test items that score high in critical thinking for national standardized tests, including HESI, NLN, NCLEX, and Excelsior College (Regents).

She was an associate editor and section editor of the Managers Forum for the Journal of Emergency Nursing for more than 10 years and is a contributing editor; section editor for the emergency section of the *American Journal of Nursing*. She has also been a legal expert/consultant in more than 45 cases.

Contributing author: June Marshall, RN, MS, CNAA,BC

June Marshall, RN, MS, CNAA,BC has been a pediatric nurse for more than 33 years, and has worked in a variety of roles including staff nurse, clinical nurse specialist, adjunct faculty, entrepreneur, and nurse administrator. She has worked in inpatient, ambulatory, rehabilitation, and home care settings. She has also lectured and served as a preceptor for undergraduate and graduate students in pediatric nursing in a variety of clinical settings.

Marshall has presented at numerous local, regional, and national conferences, has published numerous articles, and has contributed a chapter to a textbook on pediatric brain injuries. She is a member of Sigma Theta Tau and is actively involved in the local district of the Texas Nurses Association. She is also an editorial advisor for *Strategies for Nurse Managers*, published by HCPro, Inc.

Marshall has served as faculty for a nursing leadership academy and has presented a variety of organizational development topics for the participants. She also served as project director for an organization pursuing ANCC Magnet Recognition Program® designation. In 2006, she was named one of the "Great 100 Nurses" by the Texas Nurses' Association and the Dallas-Fort Worth Hospital Council.

Introduction

Critical thinking in the pediatric unit

LEARNING OBJECTIVE

After reading this section, the participant should be able to

- describe the characteristics of the pediatric unit that require good critical thinking skills

Back to basics

Whether nurses care for children in a pediatric specialty hospital or in a facility that treats primarily adult patient populations, they need to understand that children are not simply little adults. Pediatric nurses have a responsibility to understand the wide range of developmental needs that accompany each stage of life from infancy through adolescence. Critical thinking is the key to providing safe, effective nursing care for infants, children, and teens.

To be successful at mentoring and supporting critical thinking, you need to be willing to learn some basic principles involved in critical thinking. These fundamental concepts apply to all nurses, regardless of their specialty.

To make the most of this book as your resource for critical thinking, take time to review all of the content before you implement the helpful tools. It may be tempting to just start using them immediately, but you would not expect a new nurse to understand the relationship between dehydration and changes in electrolyte values in an infant without some foundational knowledge of pediatric anatomy and physiology. That same principle applies here. The tools do not provide answers: the answers lie in grasping the concepts of critical thinking.

Critical thinking and the pediatric setting

Pediatric units are places filled with "unknowns" that require nursing staff to display unique qualities and high levels of critical thinking, both as individuals and as part of a team.

The unknowns that make pediatric settings such interesting places include:

- How many patients will I have?
- Will their parents be here to help me take better care of them?
- Will my assignment be manageable?
- Do I have access to resources to address complex issues?
- Will I face parental conflict when caring for my patients?
- Do I have the skills necessary to address my patients' developmental needs?
- Will any of my patients require transfer to the ICU?

Many nurses are driven to pediatrics because of a love for children, coupled with the challenge of providing care for infants, children, and adolescents with a broad range of diagnoses. The multidisciplinary team whose members get to know one another's strengths and weaknesses quickly demonstrates good decision-making skills in providing child and family-centered care. A sense of unspoken trust usually develops among these team members, and individual team members' strengths contribute to quality patient outcomes. In this environment, the pediatric nurse needs to have all the attributes of a critical thinker, and needs to know how to use strategies that aid critical thinking to deal with patients' complex needs and multiple age groups and family systems, combined with a vast array of diagnoses.

Pediatric nurses will be faced with patients who present through a variety of points of entry including the emergency department, the operating room, and ambulatory care settings, and with an unlimited number of problems and needs. Pediatric nurses must be able to make decisions that apply to a multitude of scenarios for every age-specific patient category. Not only must these pediatric nurses have sound knowledge of normal growth and development from infancy through adolescence, they must understand a broad range of medical and surgical diagnoses. In addition, pediatric nurses must be sensitive to the needs of parents, siblings, and other family members in the face of the child's or adolescent's condition.

Pediatric nurses are also expected to manage busy patient assignments and function as effective multidisciplinary team members to meet these complex patient and family needs. This area of nursing practice requires not only critical thinking, but also intuitive judgment that comes from experience. The most successful pediatric nurses are those who possess strong critical thinking skills and can apply them for effective decision-making. Clearly, this level of experience is something that new graduate nurses are not prepared for without extensive training and work experience in pediatric settings.

The three main areas in which pediatric nurses apply critical thinking skills are admission, treatment, and discharge.

Admission

The admission process is a critical point in the child's hospitalization. Key facts gathered during the initial assessment help chart the course for all team members that subsequently provide care for this pediatric patient. Careful documentation of the child's history of present illness, past health history, growth and developmental status, and important family issues and concerns can assist the nurse in developing a plan of care that will address identified problems and best meet the child's and family's needs.

Critical thinking is essential to help the nurse view the big picture of the child's illness and family system and the impact on the hospitalization and treatment plan. During this admission period, the pediatric nurse also uses these critical thinking skills to identify, anticipate, and prioritize the patient's and family's needs based upon the child's diagnosis and current condition, as well as the family's issues, concerns, and coping mechanisms.

Attributes of critical thinking during the admission process

The following examples demonstrate application of the concepts and approaches of critical thinking at this entry point of pediatric inpatient care. Strategies and attributes of critical thinking during the admission process include the following abilities:

Independent thinker

- Identifies and initiates appropriate interventions based on assessment findings and knowledge of the child's diagnosis or condition.

- Recognizes when patient assignments require additional personnel to provide safe care, facilitate efficient patient throughput, and make the unit run smoothly.

Evaluates evidence and facts

- Upon admission, the parent states the child has been congested and is irritable and vomiting and hasn't eaten solid foods in two days. The child's temperature is 103 degrees Fahrenheit.

Explores consequences before making decisions or taking action

- The nurse knows the resident on call is busy in the emergency department seeing other patients and that it will be at least an hour before the child will be evaluated and the admission orders written.

Evaluates policy

- The nurse recognizes that although the physician will be delayed in seeing the patient, there are some initial interventions the RN can implement to make the child more comfortable until the doctor arrives. The RN contacts the physician by phone to obtain a verbal order for an antipyretic and informs the charge nurse of the patient's condition.

Confident in decisions

- Knowing that the patient has not been tolerating oral liquids, the RN requests the physician to order an alternate route for the medication.

Asks pertinent questions

- Understands that no assumptions should be made on admission. Despite the report given by the RN from the emergency department, the admitting nurse reviews the history with the mother to determine accuracy and ensure that all the details of the child's illness are documented in the assessment.

- Asks the parent what medicine and dose the child was given for the fever and when it was last given.

Displays curiosity

- Before the end of the shift, reads the physician's admission note and checks the patient's laboratory results.

Rejects incorrect information

- Despite the fact that the mother believes the child is more comfortable and should have something to eat now, the pediatric nurse observes the child is still gagging when awakened and encourages the mom to let the IV fluids and medications take effect before the child is given anything to drink or eat.

Treatment

Once children are admitted to the hospital and the treatment process begins, nurses are presented with a new set of challenges with multiple patient assignments and varying levels of patient acuity. With shortened lengths of stay, the need to facilitate patient throughput presents the critical thinker with the opportunity to demonstrate the ability to make decisions in a fast-paced environment. During this phase of pediatric care, nurses are more involved as a team of critical thinkers working together, contributing decision-making statements to physicians and other team members that lead to safe patient care and improved outcomes. Typically, a nurse serves in the role of charge or team leader to ensure the effective management of patient care and staff resources. Collaborative relationships with the medical staff provide opportunities for nurses to increase their clinical knowledge and impact their ability to think critically and make good patient care decisions.

Introduction

Attributes of critical thinking during treatment

Strategies and attributes of critical thinking during the treatment phase include the following abilities:

Independent thinker

- Prioritizes which patient situation requires urgent attention.

- Recognizes the need to call the pharmacy to ensure two IV medications ordered for the patient are compatible.

Evaluates evidence and facts

- Notes critical lab values, reassesses patient, and approaches provider with information and a request for orders.

Explores consequences before making decisions or taking action

- Patient's family is requesting fluids/food for an adolescent patient who is being evaluated for abdominal pain. Knowing that patients who may require surgery should be NPO, reviews lab and x-ray results with physician and communicates to patient and family that no oral intake is permitted at present.

Evaluates policy

- Mother requests that patient's father (from whom she is divorced, but who shares joint custody of this child) should not be notified of the hospital admission for a skull fracture. Nurse refers to hospital policy requiring informed consent of minor children to determine the course of action and contacts a social worker to speak with the mother about the social situation.

Confident in decisions

- During a resuscitative effort, a physician orders a dose of medication that is twice the dose recommended by the American Heart Association for Pediatric Advanced Life Support. Despite the urgent needs of the patient, the nurse reads the order back to the physician and questions the dose.

Asks pertinent questions

- The nurse is comfortable saying, "This patient's work in breathing seems increased to me since my assessment an hour ago. Would you like for me to call radiology and get them to come up and do a stat chest x-ray while you are on your way to reevaluate the patient?"

Displays curiosity

- When caring for a child with asthma who has had repeated admissions to this unit, the nurse approaches the provider and, while updating him or her on the patient's status, inquires, "Do you know anything about the new treatment protocol that was published in *The Journal of Pediatrics* last month? I read the article last week, but have never seen it implemented in our facility. Are you willing to take a look at it? This child does not seem to respond well to what we have been doing for him. This is his third admission in the past couple of months."

Rejects incorrect information

- When reviewing laboratory results, notes a three-year-old patient with diabetes has dangerously low blood sugar after her morning dose of insulin. After re-evaluating the patient, the nurse performs a finger-stick glucose test and finds the patient to have slightly elevated blood sugar. Upon discussion with the lab, the lab reported a mistake in the medical record number and that the results reported belonged to a patient in the clinic with the same first and last name.

Discharge

After receiving treatment, the options for where a patient goes next include:

- Discharge home
- Transferred to another acute care facility
- Transferred to the ICU/NICU
- Transferred to another unit within the facility
- Admitted to a rehabilitation facility
- Referred to dentist or primary care physician's office for follow-up
- Transferred to skilled nursing facility

- Discharged to juvenile detention facility
- Sent to the morgue

With more patients waiting for an empty room, there is always a push to move patients out of the unit as efficiently as we can. Nurses feel pressure as they try to ensure all the admission/transfer/discharge criteria are met for each patient. This is an additional obstacle for nurses trying to employ critical thinking as they work with the team to discharge patients to the appropriate setting. With so many risk-management and follow-up details to consider, nurses may at times overlook some details in such fast-paced environments.

As part of the discharge process, nurses need to consider the following:

- Reevaluate vital signs, pain status, neurological status

- Review documentation to ensure completeness and thoroughness

- Patients with limited English proficiency will require translation services to understand discharge instructions

- Some discharge instructions are complex and lengthy

- Time is needed to await parent/guardian to review discharge information and provide transportation home for patient

- Admissions being held on the unit that require ongoing nursing assessments and treatment after the patient is discharged

Pediatric nurses are expected to balance a number of complex tasks on busy inpatient units. They are often admitting and discharging a number of patients during the course of a shift. While balancing routine patient assignments, one or two critical incidents can demand the nurse's attention, upset the flow, and make routine aspects of care more challenging to accomplish during the course of the shift. Management must ensure these nurses have the time and resources they need to accomplish safe and effective patient care with all the elements of critical thinking, sound clinical interventions, and thorough documentation.

Attributes of critical thinking during discharge

Strategies and attributes of critical thinking during the discharge process include the following abilities:

Independent thinker

- Recognizes the discharge orders from the provider are premature and the patient will need to wait for an evaluation by one of the pulmonary consultants.

Evaluates evidence and facts

- Although parent claims "I can handle this by myself," nurse notes parent is unable to demonstrate all aspects of nasogastric tube feeding. Suggests to provider that the parent be provided additional education and home care follow-up for nasogastric feeding of the child.

Explores consequences before making decisions or taking action

- Asks who will be providing/supervising respiratory treatments for the child in the school setting.

Confident in decisions

- Although a particular dressing is ordered for the patient's scald burns, the nurse recognizes the fragile skin of the infant and suggests another option that will not require tape on the patient's skin.

Asks pertinent questions

- Asks adolescent patient whose parents both work evening shifts, "Is there someone who can help you with these dressing changes in the afternoon when you get home from school?"

Displays curiosity

- While holding a patient being admitted for cystic fibrosis, the nurse asks the physician about the clues that led to this diagnosis.

Listens to others and is able to give feedback

- Makes sure the new parents understand the discharge instructions for their eight-day-old newborn by asking them to repeat them back. The pediatric nurse has the parents demonstrate the correct method of administering oral medications and checking the baby's temperature.

Encouraging the development of critical thinking in pediatric nurses

Much of the critical thinking needed in the pediatric setting comes from work experiences and specific patient/family scenarios that nurses "bookmark" in their minds. All pediatric nurses should be actively involved in the orientation and development of both new graduate nurses and experienced adult nurses who join the pediatric setting. Without passing along these book-marked events, we cannot help others to develop their critical thinking capabilities.

We want pediatric nurses who are able to

- recognize a problem
- know what to do
- know when to do it
- know how to do it
- know why they are doing it

Pediatric nurses know what outcomes they want for each patient and recognize how their nursing judgment and skills affect these outcomes. Recognizing the role critical thinking plays in achieving desired patient outcomes is the first step to creating and achieving an environment that promotes sound clinical judgments.

To promote critical thinking in pediatric settings, incorporate the ANA *Scope and Standards of Pediatric Nursing Practice* in the process of orientation and ongoing development by having all staff sign a commitment to these practice standards. Clearly communicate to all nurses what is expected of them regarding their abilities in decision-making, and then promote and encourage their ongoing development.

It takes a special person to be a pediatric nurse. Being a pediatric nurse at the side of a patient and family when they face crises, are vulnerable, and are in need of medical/nursing care is a privilege. Along with that privilege comes tremendous responsibility and the power to make a difference in the lives of families entrusting their child's care to us.

References

ANA. 2003. *Scope and Standards of Pediatric Nursing Practice*. Washington, DC: American Nurses Publishing.

Cohen, Shelley. 2006. *Critical Thinking in the Emergency Department: Skills to Assess, Analyze, and Act*. Marblehead, MA: HCPro, Inc.

Chapter 1

Defining critical thinking

By Polly Gerber Zimmermann, RN, MS, MBA, CEN

LEARNING OBJECTIVES

After reading this section, the participant should be able to

- identify key aspects of critical thinking
- explain how nurses develop competency in critical thinking

Why critical thinking?

For educators and nurse leaders, critical thinking is like the weather: Everybody is talking about it, but nobody seems to know what to do about it. Passing the NCLEX only validates that new graduates have the *minimal* amount of knowledge needed to provide safe nursing care. Application of clinical critical thinking and judgment is at the heart of what makes a healthcare provider *nurse* (as a verb) compared to being a technician who completes tasks by rote. Critical thinking is at the core of safe nursing practice, and thus encouraging its development in every nurse should be an aim for all educators.

Becoming a professional nurse

Nursing is a hands-on profession for which clinical experience plays a crucial role in professional development. Nurses have to progress through various levels before they reach proficiency. Managers and educators need to appreciate that new graduate nurses are at a different level, with different needs, than experienced nurses in their professional critical thinking.

Benner's stages of growth

Benner (1984) is well known for identifying and describing the five stages through which nurses proceed in their professional growth. Benner's stages are

Beginner: Has little experience and skills, learning by rote, completing education requirements.

Advanced beginner: Can perform adequately with some judgment, usually at this stage upon graduation.

Competent: Able to foresee long-range goals and are mastering skills. Still lack the experience to make instantaneous decisions based on intuition. Most nurses take up to one year to reach this stage.

Proficient: View situation as a whole, rather than its parts. Able to develop a solution.

Expert: Intuition and decision-making are instantaneous. Most nurses take at least five years in an area of practice to reach this stage.

So how do you take your inexperienced graduates and set them on the road to proficiency? And how do you help your more experienced nurses—who may have been practicing for years, yet you would never label them experts—reach that higher level? This book provides information, strategies, and tools to help you coach nurses at all stages of development as they hone their critical thinking skills, improve their judgment, and become better nurses. Chapter 3 discusses teaching critical thinking in a classroom setting, and other chapters include ongoing strategies for developing critical thinking in the clinical environment.

The goal in encouraging and developing critical thinking is to help nurses progress effectively through the stages of development. No one wants 10-year nurse employees who have the equivalent of one year of experience simply repeated 10 times.

So what is critical thinking?

Alfaro-LeFevre (1999) defines critical thinking as careful, deliberate, outcome-focused (results-oriented) thinking that is mastered for a context. Critical thinking is based on scientific method; the nursing process; a high level of knowledge, skills, and experience; professional standards; a positive attitude toward learning; and a code of ethics. It includes elements of constant reevaluation, self-correction, and continual striving for improvement.

Some of the characteristics of people who display critical thinking include open-mindedness, the ability to see things from more than one perspective, awareness of one's own strengths and weaknesses, and ongoing striving for improvement. The strategies commonly (and often subconsciously) used in critical thinking include reasoning (inductive reasoning, such as specific to general, or deductive reasoning, such as general to specific), pattern recognition, repetitive hypothesizing, mental representation, and intuition.

In the practical world of clinical nursing, critical thinking is the ability of nurses to see patients' needs uniquely and respond appropriately, beyond or in spite of the orders. The ability to think critically is developed through ongoing knowledge gathering, experience, reading the literature, and continuous quality improvement by reviewing one's own patient charts. An example of a nurse who displays critical thinking is when a physician orders acetaminophen (Tylenol) for a patient's fever, and the nurse questions the order because the patient has hepatitis C. A critical thinker goes beyond being a "robo-nurse" who simply does as he or she is told.

In Croskerry's study (2003), 32 types of misperceptions and biases (cognitive disposition to respond) were identified in clinical decision-making. Everyone is influenced by what they see most often, most recently, or most dramatically. Cognitive errors may be avoided by always striving to consider alternatives; by decreasing reliance on memory (instead, use cognitive aids such as reference books); by using cognitive forcing strategies, such as a protocol; by taking time to think; and by having rapid and reliable feedback and follow-up to avoid repeating errors.

The overarching goal is to help shorten new graduate nurses' on-the-job learning curve, and give directed assistance to all nurses in their critical thinking development.

Del Bueno's definition of critical thinking

There are many definitions of critical thinking, and one of the most helpful is Dorothy Del Bueno's Performance-Based Development System. Del Bueno determined that nursing competency involves three skills: interpersonal skills, technical skills, and critical thinking.

Del Bueno defines critical thinking in a clinical setting with the following four aspects:

- Can the nurse recognize the patient's problem?
- Can the nurse safely and effectively manage the problem?
- Does the nurse have a relative sense of urgency?
- Does the nurse do the right thing for the right reason?

Del Bueno discussed an example from her work on responses to a taped scenario of a one-day postop trauma patient. On the tape shown to nurses, the patient suddenly becomes diaphoretic, pale, short of breath with tachypnea, and holds the right side of the chest, complaining of pain. An ABG result is given showing respiratory alkalosis. The expectation is that nurses will recognize this is a potential pulmonary embolism or pneumothorax (an alteration in respiration), manage the patient with oxygen, assess breath sounds, raise the head of the bed, call the physician, etc. And experienced nurses should anticipate physician orders, such as a portable chest x-ray or an EKG. But Del Bueno found that 75% of inexperienced and 25% of experienced nurses said they would manage the patient's alkalosis by *only* having the patient breathe into a paper bag.

Overall, she found that only 25%–30% of inexperienced nurses (less than one year of clinical experience) had acceptable results. The range of acceptable results was from 12% to 60%, and there was no difference between nurses' performance based on their educational preparation and/or whether they had previous healthcare experience (such as being a technician or an LPN). She found that 65% of experienced nurses had acceptable results, and that the number was higher (85%) in some specialties. Overall, she found that nurses' greatest limitations were in recognition and management of renal and neurological problems.

References

Alfaro-LeFevre, R. 1999. *Critical Thinking in Nursing: A Practical Approach.* Philadelphia: WB Saunders.

Benner P. 1984. *From Novice to Expert.* Menlo Park, CA: Addison-Wesley.

Brown, S. 2000. "Shock of the new." *Nursing Times* 96 (38): 27.

Charnley, E. 1999. "Occupational stress in the newly qualified staff nurse." *Nursing Standard* 13 (29): 32–37.

Croskerry, P. 2003. "The importance of cognitive errors in diagnosis and strategies to minimize them." *Academy of Medicine* 78 (8): 775–780.

Del Bueno, D. 2001. "Buyer beware: The cost of competence." *Nursing Economics* 19 (6): 259–257.

Gries, M. 2000. "Don't leave grads lost at sea." *Nursing Spectrum.* Accessed on July 27, 2006 from *http://community.nursingspectrum.com/MagazineArticles/article.cfm?AID=800.*

Huber, D. 2000. *Leadership and Nursing Care Management,* 2nd ed. Philadelphia: WB Saunders.

Norris, T. L. 2005. "Making the transition from student to professional nurse." In B. Cherry and S. R. Jacob, *Contemporary Nursing: Issues, Trends, & Management,* 3rd ed. St. Louis: Elsevier/Mosby.

Tingle, C. A. 2000. "Workplace advocacy as a transition tool." *LSNA Insider.* June.

Zimmermann, P. G. 2002. "Guiding principles at triage: Advice for new triage nurses." *Journal of Emergency Nursing* 28 (1): 24–33.

Zimmerman, P. G., and R. D. Herr. 2006. *Triage Nursing Secrets.* St. Louis: Elsevier/Mosby.

©2007 HCPro, Inc.

New graduate nurses and critical thinking

By Polly Gerber Zimmermann, RN, MS, MBA, CEN

LEARNING OBJECTIVES

After reading this section, the participant should be able to

- analyze the factors that contribute to new graduates' lack of critical thinking
- identify strategies to facilitate critical thinking in new graduates

Why don't new graduates think critically?

Educators' and nurse leaders' desire to develop nurses' critical thinking is undoubtedly more pressing for new graduate nurses. You may wonder why these nurses, who have just completed their education, do not display the qualities and skills you either expect or want. It's important to understand that new graduates face many stresses as they transition from students to registered nurses, and these stresses impede their ability to learn and progress.

Stresses for new graduate nurses

Charnley (1999) identified four categories that lead to stress in novice nurses:

1. **Reality of practice:** They think they are supposed to have all the answers, are overwhelmed by the volume of work, and feel guilty because they cannot spend more time with patients.

2. **Unfamiliarity with the structure of the organization:** They spend valuable time looking for supplies.

3. **Lack of professional relationships:** They lack an understanding of the roles of health-care providers, and their dependence on other staff may cause anxiety. They often lack mentors and support people.

4. **Lack of clinical judgment:** They have decreased confidence in their skills and decision-making abilities. This leads to apprehension.

Other special needs of new graduates have been identified, including the following (Brown, 2000; Charnley, 1999; Gries, 2000; Huber, 2000; Tingle, 2000):

Interpersonal skills/communication: They struggle with interactions with other providers in making rounds, clarifying orders, and interdisciplinary team conferences. They may miss some communication or instruction from an experienced nurse because they don't understand what the routine or slang involves. For example, one unit may refer to a septic workup as "culturing every hole." The new graduate does not understand that this standard order set includes blood cultures x2, sputum culture, urine culture, and stool culture.

Clinical: Though new nurses possess the clinical knowledge, they lack the experience that increases effectiveness, efficiency, and correctness.

Organization: This includes organization of skills and the day, often exacerbated by feeling overwhelmed and unsure how to prioritize.

Delegation: New nurses often feel uncomfortable delegating to more experienced and/or older assistants. This is exacerbated by a lack of leadership skills and trust/personal knowledge of the assistants.

Priority setting: Initially, there is a tendency to focus on tasks, rather than critical thinking planning.

Assertiveness: There can be hesitancy to say no or to understand the difference between being assertive and being aggressive.

As outlined above, the transition into practice includes a lot of stress. But new graduates can be helped to overcome the stressors and grow in critical thinking more easily when the orientation process recognizes and deals with these stresses.

Strategies to minimize stress

There are aspects you can add to orientation and for ongoing use that will minimize these stressors for new graduates. Possibilities include:

- Holding regular support group meetings with fellow orientees.

- Using a mentor or assigning a buddy (or sponsor) who builds a relationship and will follow the nurse for at least a year.

- Holding a treasure hunt for supplies or other departments during their first week of work. It will help their confidence if they know where the laboratory is located when someone stops them in the hall to ask.

- Holding a roundtable of the institution's staff nurses who have been out of school for two to five years, who can offer tips and support. (These nurses will be experienced enough to have learned, but not so experienced to have forgotten.)

- Spending a day rounding with a teaching physician who frequently admits to the unit.

- Emphasizing the importance of just "tell somebody" when something is abnormal, even if they do not know the cause or the solution. Alerting someone else will help new nurses learn. Make clear that waiting, assessing, and hoping is not a good solution.

New graduates' levels of development

When learning a new field, there are four classic stages through which the person proceeds:

- Unconsciously incompetent
- Consciously incompetent
- Consciously competent
- Unconsciously competent

The most dangerous situation is when nurses do not realize what they do not know. The best orientee is the one who realizes when to ask for help. Surprisingly, weaker students are frequently very confident, in part because they don't grasp how much there is to learn or the potential risks.

A contributing factor to this phenomenon is that newer nurses are often placed on the off shifts with other inexperienced nurses. This can limit their exposure to more-experienced nurses and they do not realize their deficiencies since their coworkers have similar levels of knowledge and judgment.

Part of developing critical thinking and orientees' ongoing self-knowledge should include encouraging them to think about "In what areas do I still need to grow?" Keep the issue of critical thinking and anticipation of potential patient complications in the forefront.

Prioritization

Prioritization typically is one of the most difficult aspects for new nurses to learn. They know if something is "normal" or "not normal," but struggle to know how much importance to attach to these classifications. Many educators and managers think new graduates will automatically pick up this discernment, but this often does not happen until after considerable time, exposure, and experience.

New graduates struggle to prioritize the needs within one patient, within a team of patients, and/or between patient and administration needs. It is necessary to provide rules and principles they can use until they develop and internalize their own clinical judgment and instinct.

Prioritization principles: Assessment

Many of the following concepts may seem simplistic and obvious, but remember that experienced nurses often forget what they, as new graduates, didn't know. Discuss the following aspects in a critical-thinking class, and include them during orientation and throughout new graduates' initial development:

Review Maslow's Hierarchy of Needs and ABCD: While familiar content, many new graduates have not specifically identified that "D for disability" includes mental status/level of consciousness (LOC), neurological and motor function, and pain. Pain, while not a good thing, is not always the worst thing. Sometimes in an effort to overcompensate for the past when analgesia received inadequate attention, pain is given almost absolute priority in the nursing curriculum.

Two common areas of weakness in new graduates are failure to ask all aspects of a pain assessment (PQRST) and failure to note the severity within the ABCD prioritization. Use examples where the type of pain and/or location, rather than severity, alerts the nurse to the problem, such as a substernal pressure that the patient rates as a 5. Use examples in which the severity matters: a significant shock (Circulation) takes priority over a mild wheezing (Breathing).

Onset (sudden over gradual): True sudden onset of symptoms can signal a catastrophic event. It is a true "sudden" onset if the patient can recall the exact time or activity when it began, and the maximum intensity is reached immediately (in less than one minute).

Actual over potential: A common error of new graduates is to focus on a "more important" potential future problem than what is currently going on. For instance, they assume the asthmatic patient who states he or she will stop his or her prednisone will take priority over someone who is currently experiencing low blood pressure. Emphasize first things first: Treat actual problems before preventing a future one.

Systemic over local (life before limb): Something that has a systemic implication, or involves multiple systems, is a priority. If no other access can be obtained, an IV is started in the leg to administer the medication to stop continuous statis epilepticus.

Trends: A trend, as opposed to an isolated incident, could be an indication of something more serious. Trends include a steady progressive decline, minor symptoms that recur repeatedly or increase in severity, and/or symptoms that are associated with other definitive (especially systemic) changes.

Compared to the patient's normal: Recognition of the same significant symptoms ("This is like the last time I had a kidney stone") or identification of a new distinction ("This is different from any other headache I had before") is important. When the complaint is "ordinary," such as a headache, remember there must be a reason why the patient thought it was important enough to report. Always consider the caregivers' perception of changes in the patient, as they know the person better than anyone.

For example, one geriatric patient was reassured by three nurses that her reported urinary incontinence was "typical" for the elderly. It took the fourth nurse to assess this symptom as a new onset, with urinary burning, and take the necessary actions to diagnose the patient's new urinary tract infection.

Patient demographics: Certain groups are more vulnerable for rapid worsening or atypical symptoms and should receive more consideration. This includes the immunosuppressed, whether by age (the very young and the very old), medication (steroid administration), disease (diabetes mellitus, HIV/AIDS), or past history (splenectomy, donor organ recipient). Similarly, greater concern should be given to patients with multiple comorbidities (their systems are already taxed for coping and will be more easily overwhelmed), or a history of the "worst-case scenario" in the past for these symptoms (e.g., "This is just like I felt when I had my heart attack").

Prioritization principles: Time management

Medications tend to be a priority and new graduates should be encouraged to consider the type and timing of medications. Anti-diabetic medications and antibiotics are usually given priority because of the consequences if they are not given in a timely manner. If two antibiotics are ordered for the same time, give the one with the shortest interval until the next dose first.

In school, nursing assessment and teaching are emphasized. The reality is that most hospitalized patients have a "diagnosis" and one of nursing's main functions is to properly administer the treatments prescribed for the patient's improvement. Why is the patient here? Make sure the "cures" are being administered.

Prioritization principles: Administrative

Patients before paperwork: Students from a heavily regulated industry, such as licensed practical nurses who worked in long-term care facilities, or those who truly understand legal implications, tend to overemphasize the documentation. Remind them that "post" charting is allowed if identified as such.

Stop any harm immediately: Those inexperienced in leadership tend to focus on others dealing with problems rather than directly taking care of it themselves. If an aide is making an error, go in and correct it now rather than telling the charge nurse, asking for more inservices, writing up an incident report, or even speaking to the aide at the end of the shift.

WHAT rather than WHO: An inexperienced nurse is likely to be intimidated and respond first to an authority figure who is barking orders. A serious patient need is always first. Have them role-play stating, "I must take care of this first, then I can be back and talk with you in about a minute."

Remind learners when talking about prioritization that everyone does receive care even if they are not first. Prioritization just recognizes that one person can only do so much at a time and there are competing demands. Prioritization involves the right care to the right person at the right time for the right reason.

Identifying worst-case scenarios, stereotypes, and expected abnormal findings

Worst-case scenarios

Another significant area in which new graduates need help is identifying and ruling out the worst-case scenario that could happen with a complaint. People make decisions heavily influenced by what they experience most often, most recently, or most dramatically in relation to the current situation. New graduates have mainly been exposed to textbook stable cases in clinical experiences.

Give new graduates examples and specifically identify what would be the worst complication. Ask them how they would know the worst-case scenario was occurring when dealing with any patient, condition, or scenario. The one-day postoperative patient may be restless due to pain, but has shock been ruled out? How would you do that? This is particularly important to stress during a critical-thinking class, but it should also be brought up again and again. Remember, repetition is the mother of all learning. New graduates should know that for each patient they take care of, they should first think, "What is the worst-case scenario?" so that this may be ruled out as necessary, and the process should eventually become automatic.

There is a familiar phrase used in medicine, "When you hear hoofbeats, think horses, not zebras." It illustrates the overarching principle that nurses should first consider the most common causes for a patient's presentation, but be alert to the fact there are some "zebras" out there. Don't miss them.

Stereotypes

It can be helpful to include common misconceptions (which are often subconscious) in illustrations. For example, common stereotypes may include that psychiatric patients don't have physical problems, or that all old people are a little bit confused. Nurses should ascertain whether the elderly patient with new-onset confusion has low glucose, low pulse-oximeter reading, or a urinary tract infection. False assumptions can lead to a wrong action.

Expected abnormal findings

What is an expected finding for this given condition? Make the distinction that significant "abnormal" findings are not a concern when they are a part of that patient's known medical condition. It is not alarming that a patient with pneumonia admitted for intravenous antibiotics has an elevated white blood cell count (WBC). It is more necessary to know if the WBC is higher, lower, or the same since starting the antibiotics. Similarly, it is not alarming that the patient with pancreatitis has amylase and lipase levels three times the normal value—that is how the diagnosis is made. It is more important to rule out serious complications such as hypocalcemia, hypovolemia, hypoxia, or severe pain.

Ongoing development

Awareness is the first step toward beginning to change behavior. Orientation often focuses on "how we do things here," and includes forms, policies, and the mission statement.

Orientation also should include a purposeful identification and focus on critical thinking. Discussion should include making clinical correlations, applying them to each patient's unique presentation, understanding the reason things are being done, and focusing on the most essential aspects in the proper order. Bringing these types of approaches to the forefront will help the new graduate understand what is needed to succeed.

References

Alfaro-LeFevre, R. 1999. *Critical Thinking in Nursing: A Practical Approach*. Philadelphia: WB Saunders.

Benner, P. 1984. *From Novice to Expert*. Menlo Park, CA: Addison-Wesley.

Brown, S. 2000. "Shock of the new." *Nursing Times* 96 (38): 27.

Charnley, E. 1999. "Occupational stress in the newly qualified staff nurse." *Nursing Standard* 13 (29): 32–37.

Croskerry, P. 2003. "The importance of cognitive errors in diagnosis and strategies to minimize them." *Academy of Medicine* 78 (8): 775–780.

Del Bueno, D. 2001. "Buyer beware: The cost of competence." *Nursing Economics* 19 (6): 259–257.

Gries, M. 2000. "Don't leave grads lost at sea." *Nursing Spectrum*. Accessed on July 27, 2006 from *http://community.nursingspectrum.com/MagazineArticles/article.cfm?AID=800*.

Huber, D. 2000. *Leadership and Nursing Care Management*, 2nd ed. Philadelphia: WB Saunders.

Norris, T. L. 2005. "Making the transition from student to professional nurse." In B. Cherry and S. R. Jacob, *Contemporary Nursing: Issues, Trends, & Management*, 3rd ed. St. Louis: Elsevier/Mosby.

Tingle, C. A. 2000. "Workplace advocacy as a transition tool." *LSNA Insider* (June).

Zimmermann, P. G. 2002. "Guiding principles at triage: Advice for new triage nurses." *Journal of Emergency Nursing* 28 (1): 24–33.

Zimmerman, P. G. and R. D. Herr. 2006. *Triage Nursing Secrets*. St. Louis: Elsevier/Mosby.

The critical thinking classroom

By Polly Gerber Zimmermann, RN, MS, MBA, CEN

LEARNING OBJECTIVE

After reading this section, the participant should be able to

- determine classroom strategies to teach, promote, and support the development of critical thinking

Critical thinking can be taught

The tendency is to view critical thinking as an abstract formula to memorize. Rather, it is a process of applying acquired textbook knowledge to the clinical setting and specific patients. All nurses usually need some initial assistance in applying their knowledge to the situation, particularly for high-volume, high-risk, or infrequent patient presentations with which they have had little familiarity during their education or experience.

Classes that discuss and teach critical thinking can be beneficial for both new graduates and more experienced nurses. New graduates and new hires will benefit from classes held during orientation, but it also may be useful to periodically schedule general-attendance classes so that other nurses may participate.

Background preparation

Teacher preparation

Educators can tend to spend excessive energy on "what" to teach. Just as important is "how" to teach—determining the best way to communicate the information so learning takes place. When planning an educational session, focus less on "What am I going to say today?" and more on "What are my listeners going to learn today?"

Teaching is not pouring wisdom into passive listeners. The teacher is a guide for active participation through a learning experience. Watch the audience's responses. That is the only way to perceive the need to repeat material, vary the presentation, or illustrate the content's application for this group.

Consider the learner's motivation

Why will attendees be motivated to learn? The driving force for all ordinary behavior is "What's in it for me?" Avoid the "Field of Dreams" approach—i.e., if we plan it, they will come and learn. Instead, use the human tendency toward selfishness—what's in it for me?—to teaching's advantage. Further breaking down that number one motivation reveals the three main aspects people want from education sessions. People want to

- get something accomplished/meet their goals
- receive personal recognition, power, or influence
- have social interaction and enjoyment

Most of us are usually more influenced by one factor than another, but there are aspects of all three in everyone. Time spent in the classroom should meet all three purposes. Give certificates; have checklists to complete; give personal, positive, public praise; and add humor or games.

Generational differences

Understanding motivational aspects is important when considering today's multigenerational work force. Everyone is influenced by the time in which they were raised, when they developed their mindset, values, priorities, and styles. As the Arab proverb says, "People resemble their times more than they resemble their parents."

Baby Boomers are individuals born between 1946–1964. The average age for registered nurses is 44 to 47 years. Baby Boomers are more likely to act out of a sense of duty and a drive to accomplish.

Generation Xers are those born between 1965–1980. They want independence and flexibility; they want to know "Why?" (as they focus on results); and they want fun. If an activity is not worthwhile to them, they do not feel a sense of obligation to stick it out and will check out physically and/or mentally.

Generation Y is the generation born between 1981–2006. They are entering the workplace with high expectations for themselves, their employers, and their managers, and expect coaching, training, and support to help them achieve their goals.

Many educators fall into the Baby Boomer age category, whereas new graduate nurses often fall into the Generation X or Generation Y categories. Remember that approaches used for the established work force, or even for you when you were a new graduate, may not work now. It's important to tailor learning experiences to meet the needs of all generations in your classes.

Professional nurses' goals

David Shore (1997) defined what professionals want from their educational offerings: They want to be an ACE. Specifically, they expect *Access* (to peers, resources, and networking), *Credentialing* (external validation of what they know and whether it is still correct), and *Education* (information to make a demonstrable, practical difference in their practice).

Keep these expectations in mind when planning learning experiences. Also note that experienced nurses are very interested in regulations (e.g., "The Joint Commission requires . . . ") or legal requirements (e.g., "In this case, a nurse was sued for . . . ").

Setting the stage

Classroom environment

The classroom environment plays a key role in your critical-thinking course. Create an atmosphere that awakens the participant's whole brain and senses. Communicate, even on a subconscious level, that this is an enjoyable, desirable place and activity.

Seating: As much as possible, use a half-circle for small groups, and a fishbone configuration for larger groups. Avoid having a group at a table with stragglers in the row behind. Avoid hiders: participation is necessary for learning.

Use color: One study found that visual aids with color and symbols increased long-term retention by 14–38%.

Peripheral learning: We use sight for 75% of our learning. While we speak at 125 words per minute, we think at about 600 words per minute. Give the learner something to do with the extra 475-word capacity. When their mind or eyes start to drift, let them fall on educational posters.

If it is a dedicated classroom, make posters that specifically apply to the content that is being taught. If it is a generic classroom, use prevention and healthcare associations' free posters—then even the housekeeping staff learns.

Music: Play upbeat music before class, during breaks, and after class. Baroque is recommended because it matches the rhythm of the heart and enhances learning. Use lively pop music with a distinct beat you can dance to—it will pump up the energy in the room.

Frequent breaks: Experts recommend taking a five-minute "exercise" break every 40–50 minutes, but it's even more effective to take a one-minute break every 25 minutes or so. Set a kitchen timer and, when it dings, announce that it's time for a break and turn on the music. Encourage general arm stretching, walking around, etc. Indicate participation is optional.

After one minute, turn off the music and start class, usually with a joke. These breaks should be in addition to the scheduled longer break midway through the class. Teachers fear these breaks will create a loss of control of the classroom but that does not happen with adults when done with purposeful actions and explanations. Many students indicate "the music break" was one of their favorite aspects of the class.

There are many reasons to take these frequent breaks. Necessary bathroom breaks are then quickly facilitated without disrupting the classroom—and those who straggle back in miss the reward of humor. Exercise increases cognitive functioning, attention, and alertness. It pulls in the kinesthetic learners and individuals who have minor attention-deficit problems.

However, the real purpose for the breaks is to aid learning. People remember the first and the last things—educators call this the primacy and recency effect. More breaks mean more "firsts" and "lasts" to make an impression on one's brain.

Classroom content

New graduate content

When new graduates are asked about their biggest fears and concerns, they mention concerns about how to handle their many responsibilities (during school they only had to deal with one or two patients), how to handle emergencies (especially a "code"), and how to communicate with physicians / when to call the doctor.

The first step in teaching critical thinking may be to help them develop a plan of action to enable more effective responses when encountering these issues in practice. This will free up their energy to allow them to focus on the subtle patient-care assessments and important interventions.

Use some of these tips as a starting point for discussion.

Getting work done

- Provide a cheat sheet form for taking report or for the day's organization.

- Set "drop dead" times within your day (such as "all 9 a.m. medications to be in the patients' bodies by 9:30 a.m.") as guideposts for your progress in the day's time management.

- Work ahead. Always assume the unexpected will happen—it does.

- Keep current with your charting. It is harder to recall everything at the end of the day.

- Constantly reprioritize. Don't ask yourself, "What are all the things I should do?" but "What is most important for me to do?"

Emergencies/code

- Get help. For a code, if nothing else, go out in the hall and say, "I need help right now in room X!" in an urgent tone, with a loud, calm voice.

- Memorize the Institute for Healthcare Improvement (IHI) or other guidelines for activating a Rapid Response Team (see reference in resources section of Chapter 9). The IHI and other organizations have established recognized criteria for dealing with patients who could be critical and deteriorating. If anyone criticizes being contacted, cite the higher authority. "Well, the IHI indicates a Rapid Response Team should be activated for a sustained blood pressure below 90 systolic, so I felt it was advisable to follow the national criteria and get additional assistance."

Contacting the physician

- Take the initiative and introduce yourself to the physicians who admit frequently to your unit.

- Rehearse introductory statements/scripts for common needs. "Your patient (name) in room X is reporting Y and requesting Z. Do you want to order anything at this time?"

General advice

- Be slow to join a clique

- Make friends with the unit secretary

- Make your rounds during the night whether others do or not

- Make your own list of procedures or skills you have never experienced and let everyone on the unit (especially during orientation) know your desire to watch/participate in these tasks.

Teach in the context of clinical application

When planning a critical-thinking class for new graduates, experienced nurses, or both, remember that your session will be enhanced when the classroom time is spent applying knowledge to the clinical setting. Do not simply give a theory lecture. Instead, use images from books or sample labs. For example, you could hold up a picture of purpura and ask, "What do you think when you walk in and your patient looks like this?" Or present lab results (see below) and ask which value nurses should take care of first.

Value	Result	Normals
Glucose	193 mg/dL	70–110 mg/dL
BUN	8 mg/dL	10–20 mg/dL
Cr	0.7 mg/dL	0.7–1.2 mg/dL
Sodium	131 mEq/dL	136–145 mEq/dL
Potassium	3.2 mEq/dL	3.5–5.0 mEq/dL
SGOT/ALT	1932 IU/L	13–40 IU/L
SGPT/AST	2360 IU/L	7–60 IU/L
Bilirubin total	2.9 mg/dL	0.2–1.2 mg/dL

Experienced nurses are likely to pick potassium, but new graduate nurses rarely do so. Nurses learn the importance of potassium levels, in part, from work experience. This exercise will shorten the learning curve. You can also ask additional questions, such as

- What disease does the patient have?

- How does the patient look?

- Why isn't the sodium level the most important since it is "lower" than the potassium deficiency?

Prioritization

Nurses not only need to know what to do, but the importance and order in which things should be done. Nurses of all experience levels may need help with prioritization for multiple needs within one patient, between multiple patients, and between patient and administrative needs.

 Case study: Prioritization doesn't always come naturally

At one associate-degree nursing program, the faculty had assumed students would naturally pick up the concepts of prioritization. The faculty was appalled when the students scored below the national average in this category on a standardized test.

To remedy the problem, the nursing program added classroom time to talk about principles of prioritization, which was followed by a year-long integration of such principles into future content. By giving the problem a specific focus and emphasis, the school's students now score above national average in prioritization.

The handout developed for the second-year students can be found at the end of this chapter (Figure 3.1). This tool can either be used during critical-thinking classes, or given to attendees as a take-home reminder.

Strategies to teach prioritization

One way to teach prioritization principles is to use sample test questions dealing with prioritization, followed by a discussion of the rationale. For example:

Question: It is most important for the nurse to care for which patient complaint first?

    a.   Patient with type II diabetes mellitus with an a.m. blood sugar of 190mg.

    b.   Patient with a K+ of 3.2mEq who is receiving a K+ rider IVPB and states his arm is sore.

    c.   Patient with asthma treated with high-dose steroids states he is catching the "flu"; temperature is 100.4°F (38°C).

    d.   Patient with pneumonia being treated with IV antibiotics for one day. Today's WBC is 14,000mm^3.

Answer: The intended answer is C because immunocompromised patients present with suppressed symptoms. Follow-up discussion could include the difference if A was hypoglycemic, normal side effects of potassium infusions, and the fact that D is already being treated. However, discussion should also include the need to look at trends. If this was the patient's third day on antibiotics and the WBC is the same or increasing, we need to initiate action toward consideration of changing antibiotics.

First rule out the worst-case scenario

Everyone is influenced by what he or she sees most often or most recently. When dealing with a patient presentation, nurses must learn how to rule out the most lethal possible cause first.

One way is to indicate a patient condition seen frequently on the unit or department where the nurses in the particular class work, such as a one-day postoperative hip replacement. Ask the attendees what is essential for the nurse to do today. Common responses will likely include manage the pain, check the operative dressing, assess bowel and breath sounds, check the hemoglobin, watch the IV site and urine output, and verify PT is initiated.

Next ask what are the worst-case scenarios (i.e., most lethal complication) that could happen with this patient. How would you know if the patient was having those conditions? Discuss shock (possible loss of two liters in the hip), severe anemia (requiring transfusion), aspiration pneumonia, bowel ileus, sepsis, loss of circulation to the leg, dislocation of the prostethesis, or a secondary condition (myocardial infarction). Often, just the technique of bringing known material into the nurses' conscious awareness helps the process become second nature.

Use test questions and illustrative stories

Another strategy is to use test questions related to a patient presentation, and find out whether nurses assess for the worst-case scenario.

Question: A 96-year-old patient admitted with pneumonia is found crawling out of the bed. What should nurses do first?

    a.   Assess the patient's pain level.

    b.   Obtain a pulse oximeter reading.

    c.   Call for an order for a sedative.

    d.   Apply a Posey jacket.

Answer: Before you give the correct answer, B, talk about elderly patients' inability to compensate and how the brain is the most sensitive indicator for most things (low glucose, cerebral edema, etc.) Discuss whether they would feel tempted to answer differently if the person was 50 years old. Is the stereotype about all elderly people being a little confused influencing them?

Continue the lesson with a further illustration: A student nurse was told by another nurse to restrain the elderly person, which he did, but then the student nurse checked the pulse oximeter on his own. The patient was 86%.

Another true example of the danger of assuming all elderly people are confused: An elderly patient's daughter stated her mother was more confused than usual. Though the patient's pulse oximeter was 90%, no action was taken till the patient had a small stroke the next day. Diagnostics tests then revealed a small pulmonary embolism and a new stroke caused by a second clot.

Students remember stories—use them to get your point across.

New graduate nurses and more-experienced nurses who lack critical thinking skills tend to focus on the immediate task and orders rather than what should be done in the bigger picture. They fear acts of commission, such as giving the wrong medication. In doing so, they often commit acts of omission—not doing what they should do.

To train nurses how to focus on the bigger picture, start with common situations and discuss as a group what nurses should do:

- The patient has decreased pulses in his or her leg after a knee replacement. The nurse calls the resident, who reassures the nurse that the situation is fine. What should the nurse do when obtaining the same assessment two hours later?

- The patient has neuro checks ordered every two hours. The checks have been fine for the previous eight hours. It is now 2:00 a.m. and the patient is sleeping. What should the nurse do?

Often, inexperienced nurses focus on "assessing" because they are told to assess before acting. However, emphasize the need to act when they sense through assessment that something serious is wrong. Examples of actual legal cases help illustrate this point:

- A nurse charted that the patient's pulse remained 120 all night every hour on the hour, but did nothing (until the patient coded from internal hemorrhage).

- A nurse did not wake up the patient for a neuro assessment since the ABCs were stable, and the patient had some paralysis the following morning from cauda equina.

- A patient's pulse oximeter remained 80% after the physician checked the patient at 1:00 a.m. The patient coded at 6:00 a.m. with respiratory acidosis.

State how important it is to at least tell somebody. Emphasize that it is all right if nurses do not know the etiology or what treatment should be given. Discuss options if one person doesn't respond (such as the charge nurse, a colleague, the nursing supervisor, another resident, the attending physician, etc.).

Role-play what nurses should say in such situations, and remember that a little humility can go a long way. As Sylvia Rayfield (2002) suggests, start with "Help me to understand . . . "

Classroom processes

Repetition is the mother of all learning

Regardless of the style, new material needs reinforcement, and this is especially important for new graduates, as the anxiety of being new adds to the need to hear things more than once. When you teach, say something again, in a slightly different way. Use personal anecdotes, legal cases, or even published literature to illustrate the principle, emotions, and consequences of the lesson. The repetition and variety of methods are penetrating.

Use unfolding case scenarios

This technique is another way to incorporate the process of clinical critical thinking in a class-room setting. It provides the information in staggered amounts, punctuated by questions. The following are examples you can use.

The patient is a two-day postoperative hemi-colonectomy and asks for something for pain. Ask the attendees, "What is essential for the nurse to ask?" You have already decided ahead of time that the patient will have a more atypical problem, such as cholelithiasis from the anesthesia and dehydration or bladder distention after the catheter is removed, so respond appropriately to the questions the nurses ask. Don't let the "patient" tell the learners "giveaway" symptoms. Keep going until the learners specify where the pain is and palpate a positive Murphy's sign or distended bladder.

A 40-year-old presents with chest discomfort. The "patient" should also either be a cocaine user, an atypical cardiac presentation, or a smoker on birth control with a small pulmonary embolism. Did the attendees ask about drug use, prematurely rule out cardiac etiology due to the sex and age, and/or remember to check a pulse oximeter? Remind them to use incidence and "classic" presentations to help rule in considerations, but not to absolutely rule out.

 ©2007 HCPro, Inc. **Critical Thinking in the Pediatric Unit**

Instructional approach and style

Cooperative learning

A growing trend in education is to have students teach students because "he who teaches, learns the most." One way to do this is the "think, pair, and share" exercise. Learners are given the general question and provided one minute to think about it and write down their thoughts. The task could be something like, "What are the three most important things to assess for in the first day on an abdominal postoperative patient?" or "What is something that makes it easier to delegate to an aide?"

After the minute is up, the participants then pair up and share their answers. Require each person to verbalize their thoughts to their partner, rather than just agreeing with the first person's statements. After time to share, one person is chosen as the spokesperson for the duo. Use a random selector to decide who shares, such as the person with the earliest birthday in the year, so both pay attention during the sharing.

Have the spokespeople stand and randomly select a few to repeat information from the paired sharing. Another way to change the selection is to use a version of musical chairs, passing a blown-up balloon, or have everyone stand and sit down according to certain criteria.

The advantage of a "think, pair, and share" exercise is that everyone participates. It accommodates those learners who initially need more time to think or have trouble speaking before others. They have rehearsed what they will say and can choose to enhance their response with their partners' comments. You also facilitate interaction with the material because participants must conceive it, write it, speak it, hear it, and work with it.

Multi-sensory learning

Most learning occurs through visual means, then hearing, with some touch. We all have our preferred style, but everyone will learn best when the logical left side and artistic right side of the brain are engaged.

Make sure your class varies the methods used to ensure multi-sensory learning. It's been shown that retention goes up to 50% when you hear and see something.

Effective use of discussion questions for class interaction

Throughout all discussions, pose good questions to stimulate thinking. Questions include, How does that work? What does that mean? What is the worst-case scenario here? What else do you need to know to make a decision? What makes this presentation different from the ordinary presentation? What do you want to do next? Why?

Another tip is to use silence. It can be tempting to jump in with the answer to fill the quiet (often awkward) moment that follows after a question. Train yourself to wait 10 seconds to allow time for the learners to respond. Tell the audience why you are waiting. Literally count off your fingers because 10 seconds can seem like an eternity.

It can be particularly effective to wait and not respond even when the right answer is given. This prevents learners from becoming good at reading the instructor rather than thinking about the issue. Alternatives include confirming the answer, but asking the person to defend it or to play the devil's advocate with the correct answer.

In the teaching scenarios, break the information down to what is essential, and also compare similarities or differences with a known concept. "How is this different from . . . ?"

Exude passion, as well as purpose

William Arthur Ward said, "The mediocre teacher tells. The good teacher explains. The superior teacher demonstrates. The great teacher inspires." The key behind great, effective teaching is not knowledge or methodology. It is holding a genuine passion for the material and for teaching.

When teaching, pull in emotion: We often forget what we think, but almost always remember how something made us feel. The teacher's excitement and belief about the material and its importance is infectious. The learner will either catch it or (at least) respect it.

References

Raines, C. 2002. "Managing Generation X Employees" in P. G. Zimmermann, *Nursing Management Secrets.* Philadelphia: Hanley & Belfus.

Rayfield, S., and L. Manning. 2002. *Nursing Made Insanely Easy!,* 3rd ed. Gulf Shore, AL: ICAN.

Salter, C. 2001. "16 ways to be a smarter teacher." *The Fast Company* 53: 114–126.

Shore, D. A., and P. G. Zimmerman. 1997. "Marketing your continuing education program." *Journal of Emergency Nursing* 23 (4): 363–366.

Zimmermann, P. G. and R. D. Herr. 2006. *Triage Nursing Secrets.* St. Louis: Mosby/Elsevier.

Zimmermann, P. G. 2006. "Writing effective test questions to measure triage competency: Tips for making a good triage test." *Journal of Emergency Nursing* 32 (1): 106–109.

Zimmermann, P. G. 2006. "Education and Training for Triage Nurses." In P. G. Zimmermann and R. D. Herr, *Triage Nursing Secrets.* St. Louis: Elsevier.

Zimmermann, P. G. 2003. "Orienting ED nurses to triage: Using scenario-based test-style questions to promote critical thinking." *Journal of Emergency Nursing* 29 (3): 256–258.

Zimmermann, P. G. 2003. "Some practical tips for more effective teaching." *Journal of Emergency Nursing* 29 (3): 283–286.

Zimmermann, P. G. 2002. "Guiding principles at triage: Advice for new triage nurses." *Journal of Emergency Nursing* 28 (1): 24–33.

Zimmermann, P. G. 2002. "The difference between teaching nursing students and registered nurses." *Journal of Emergency Nursing* 28 (6): 574–578.

Sources for example cases

- Legal case of the month from the Nurses Service Organization, available at *www.nso.com/case*

- Triage Column/Case Review/Clinical Educator in the *Journal of Emergency Nursing*

- Glendon, K., and D. Ulrich. 2001. *Unfolding Cases: Experiencing the Realities of Clinical Nursing Practice.* Upper Saddle River, NJ: Prentice Hall.

Figure 3.1	Teaching critical thinking—Critical thinking course content and prioritization handout

PRIORITIZATION HANDOUT

Determining the need

Two components: history and physical assessment

History

Be disciplined to be consistent and thorough. Consider using a mnemonic.

POSHPATE: History of the chief complaint (Rutenberg, C. 2000. "Telephone Triage." *American Journal of Nursing* 100(3):77-78, 80-81.)

P	Problem
O	Onset
S	Associated Symptoms
H	Previous History
P	Precipitating factors
A	Alleviating/Aggravating factors
T	Timing
E	Etiology

- Document key findings that allowed you to rule out the worst-case scenario or that made you think there was a problem.

- Compare to the patient's normal, especially for a chronic or elderly condition. ("You look like you are having a little trouble breathing. Is that how you are feeling?")

- Your concern should be heightened if the patient is concerned enough to complain about an "ordinary" condition (e.g., headache).

Figure	*Teaching critical thinking—Critical thinking*
3.1	*course content and prioritization handout (cont.)*

Assess before acting

Question: One-day postoperative patient complains of pain. Nurses should first

a. administer the ordered prn analgesic

b. assess for the presence of bowel sounds

c. obtain a description of the pain

d. check the vital signs

Answer: C. Do not assume the pain is postoperative. Postoperative patients can have MIs or cholecystitis.

Prioritization with individual patients

Maslow

Self-actualization needs

Esteem needs

Safety needs

Physiologic needs

ABCD: A before B before C before D

A Airway	If the patient is talking, the airway is intact
B Breathing	Normal respirations are quiet and effortless
C Circulation	Pink, warm, orientation r/t perfusion
D Disability	Pain
	Neurological assessment
	Mental status changes

Quick Tip: 30-2-CAN DO means patient is adequately oxygenated and perfused to allow you to proceed. (Respirations are less than 30, oriented to person and place, obeys commands.)

Among ABCD, level of severity is considered.

Figure 3.1	*Teaching critical thinking—Critical thinking course content and prioritization handout (cont.)*

Question: All of these patients complain of being short of breath. Which patient should nurses provide care to first?

    a. Patient with bronchitis who can speak phrases

    b. Patient with emphysema with a PO2 of 92% on 2L/min

    c. Patient three days post-operative with a cough productive of green phlegm

    d. Patient with asthma on whom the nurse cannot auscultate breath sounds

Answer: D

AIRWAY

Risk for airway problems

- Decreased level of consciousness
- Sedated
- Vomiting
- Allergic reactions (unpredictable progression)

Signs of airway distress

- Hoarseness (after smoke inhalation, unrelated to a cold)
- Singed nasal hairs
- Snoring respirations (tongue falling back in an unconscious patient)
- Presence of vomitus, bleeding, secretions
- Edema of the lips/mouth tissues
- Preferred position (tripod)
- Drooling in an adult (throat is too swollen to swallow spit, epiglottis)
- Dysphagia
- Abnormal signs, such as strider, burgling, "death rattle" from secretions

Assess

- Look, listen, feel
- Level of consciousness r/t oxygenation

Interventions

• Reposition

• Suction

BREATHING

Assess

• Respiration rate AND depth

• Symmetrical chest rise and fall

• Presence and quality of bilateral breath sounds

• Pulse oximeter

Signs of respiratory problems

• Increased work of breathing (nasal flaring, retractions, expiratory grunting, accessory muscle use, head bobbing)

• Paradoxical respirations

• Jugular vein distention

• Tracheal position

• Abnormal breath sounds (silent chest is the most ominous because air is not moving)

• Color, especially circumoral (cyanosis is a late sign)

• Lack of integrity in chest wall

• Speaks in words, phrases, incomplete sentences

Figure
3.1

*Teaching critical thinking—Critical thinking
course content and prioritization handout (cont.)*

Related routine aspects to assess

• Is incentive spirometer within the patient's reach? Can/does the patient use it properly and frequently enough?

• Is oxygen on properly, correct amount?

• Peak flow

• Patient's self-rating on the work of the breathing (Borg scale)

Interventions

• Position
• Oxygen
• Ventilation

CIRCULATION

Assess

• Skin color, temperature
• Perfusion through blanching, capillary refill
• Pulse: rate, rhythm characteristics

General rule of thumb: Adults with a radial pulse have $\geq$ 80 systolic (brachial $\geq$ 70; jugular $\geq$ 60); low perfusion; respiratory and heart rate increase first, before blood pressure

Blood pressure: Adults must lose about 1500cc; children about 25% of volume before hypotension onsets

---

| Figure 3.1 | Teaching critical thinking—Critical thinking course content and prioritization handout (cont.) |

Signs of circulation difficulties

- Early signs and symptoms: loss of consciousness (LOC)
- Children: loss of peripheral, then central pulses, extremity mottling
- Uncontrolled bleeding: spurting = arterial
- Distended jugular veins
- Distant heart tones
- Pitting dependent edema: pedal, sacral in a bedridden patient
- Most frequent sign of deep-vein thrombosis: unilateral extremity swelling
- Neurovascular (5 Ps)
  - Paresthesia is the early sign; nerves are more sensitive than pulse

Interventions

- IV
  - Is the site intact?
  - Is the dressing intact?
  - Is the infusion "working" at the proper rate?

- Drainage
  - Dressing dry and intact?

- Circulation devices (foot pumps, SCDs, TED hose properly applied)

DISABILITY

Assess

- Alteration of orientation x 3 (scales)
- Alertness
- Neuro checks (Glasgow Coma Scale, PERRLA, movement/strength in all extremities)
- Pain
  - Objective score.

  - PQRST.

 ©2007 HCPro, Inc.

Figure 3.1	*Teaching critical thinking—Critical thinking course content and prioritization handout (cont.)*

- Effect on normal ADL.

- More concern if the pain wakes the patient up, reaches maximum intensity in the first minute, patient can recall the exact moment it started suddenly, or is similar to the pain the patient had for a serious etiology (e.g., "This feels like the last time I had a heart attack.").

- If patient states it is the "worst pain in my life" but appears comfortable or has a minor complaint (e.g., sore throat), ask about the person's previous worst pain experience. Any experience is the worst the first time you have it. If compared to significant event, such as childbirth, kidney stone, or broken bone, then accept it.

Assessment guidelines

Consider and rule out the worst-case scenario patients could have with this complaint.

What area or problem is most likely to result with this patient's condition?

Facial surgery	Airway/breathing
Broken arm	Compartment syndrome, loss of circulation
Diabetes	Hypoglycemia, DKA, HHNK
Abdominal surgery	Dehiscence, evisceration; shock; infection; bowel obstruction

Question: Which assessment is most important for a patient with a chest tube?

a. Respiratory rate

b. Pulse rate

c. Pain level

d. Temperature

Answer: A

Figure 3.1	Teaching critical thinking—Critical thinking course content and prioritization handout (cont.)

Question: An elderly patient is four days postoperative from abdominal surgery. Today the patient has a temperature of 103.1°F (39.5°C), 104/60, 110/20. This morning's WBC results are 20,000. It is most important for nurses to

a. administer a prn antipyretic

b. monitor the vital signs every hour

c. assess for bowel sounds

d. call the physician for antibiotics

Answer: D

Go for the most common problem first. "When you hear hoof beats, think horses, not zebras."

Question: The patient presents with a forearm deformity from falling 3 hours ago. He complains of severe pain.

What is the most likely explanation? Pain from a fracture

What must be ruled out? Compartment syndrome, loss of circulation

How will you assess this? 5 Ps; passive stretching, if relief obtained from analgesic

Patients before paperwork.

Stop any procedure causing harm.

Question: While the nurse is administering an IV antibiotic, the patient becomes flushed and complains of feeling hot. The nurses should first

a. complete an Adverse Drug Reaction form

b. call the doctor for an order for an antihistamine

c. stop the infusion

d. check the client's allergic history

Answer: C

Figure	*Teaching critical thinking—Critical thinking*
3.1	*course content and prioritization handout (cont.)*

Question: The charge nurse notices the new nursing assistant placing the patient's urine Foley bag on a hook at the height of the patient's chest. What is the best response for the nurse to make?

   a. Move the bag and speak to the assistant now.

   b. Speak to the nursing assistant at the end of the shift.

   c. Discuss the need for additional inservicing with the nurse educator.

   d. Write an incident report and inform the nurse manager.

Answer: A

Medications tend to be a priority, especially for anti-diabetic and antibiotic medications because of the lack of effectiveness if not given in a timely manner.

Question: The patient is admitted from the emergency department with a diagnosis of bacterial meningitis. Which of the following orders is most important for the nurse to do first?

   a. Obtain a set of vital signs.

   b. Administer the IV antibiotic.

   c. Perform a neuro assessment

   d. Administer the prn antipyretic.

Answer: B

Consider the timing/type of medication

Two antibiotics are ordered for 1:00 p.m. One is every 24 hours, one is every 4 hours. The nurse should administer the one ordered every 4 hours first at 1:00 pm to allow for the best interval.

Figure

3.1

Teaching critical thinking—Critical thinking course content and prioritization handout (cont.)

Question: A nurse had been involved with an emergency on the patient unit and is late in administering the team's 9:00 a.m. medications. Which of the 9:00 a.m. medications is most important for the nurse to administer first?

a. Ampicillin 1000mg IVPB every 6 hours

b. Vancomycin 1 gram IVPB every 36 hours

c. Lanoxin (Digoxin) 0.125mg daily

d. Aspirin 81mg daily

Answer: A

Question: A nurse was involved with another patient's cardiac arrest and is behind schedule with medications. It is now 8:00 a.m. Which medication is most important?

a. Colace

b. Ferrous sulfate

c. Erythromycin po

d. 70/30 insulin

Answer: D

Prioritization principles

Acute before chronic.

Question: Which of the following patients is most important for the nurse to follow up with first?

a. Reports unilateral blurry central vision for one year.

b. States has a veil starting to come across the vision in one eye.

c. Yellow discharge noted from right eye, relates had it for one day.

d. Complains of itching eyes during the spring.

Answer: B

Sudden onset is usually more serious than gradual onset. Actual over potential.

 ©2007 HCPro, Inc.

| Figure 3.1 | Teaching critical thinking—Critical thinking course content and prioritization handout (cont.) |

Trends

- **Any symptom associated with other definitive changes** (e.g., not feeling well, and a fever, and feeling short of breath)

- **Any minor symptoms that tend to recur repeatedly or intensify in severity** ("nagging" cough that won't go away, smoker)

- **Steady progressive decline**

Question: Which patient with these findings is most important for the nurse to check on first?

a. Respirations: 16, 18, 20

b. Radial pulse: 80, 86, 92

c. Blood pressure: 150/80, 130/78, 110/70

d. Pulse oximeter: 99%, 97%, 96%

Answer: C

Life before limb (systemic before local).

Question: Which patient should the nurse take care of first?

a. Patient with Billroth II procedure complaining of incisional discomfort rated "6."

b. Patient with deep-vein thrombosis complaining of shortness of breath.

c. Patient with low-back pain complaining that it radiates down the right leg.

d. Patient with chronic arterial insufficiency complaining of leg pain while walking.

Answer: B

| Figure 3.1 | Teaching critical thinking—Critical thinking course content and prioritization handout (cont.) |

Patient demographics

Presence of other risk factors increase this patient's priority

- Elderly (decreased immunity, decreased reserves to fight other stresses)
- Very young (decreased immunity)
- Altered immunity (leukemia, HIV+ or AIDS, taking steroids, splenectomy)
- Transplanted organs (risk of electrolyte imbalance, immunosuppressed)
- Multiple comorbidities (especially diabetes because less immunity)
- Pregnancy (risk to fetus)
- Reaction that has a potential to worsen (overdose, allergic response)

Avoid exposure of susceptible individuals.

Question: The unit will receive a new admission from the emergency department diagnosed with bacterial pneumonia. Which of the following patients would be the best choice for a roommate?

a. 19-year-old with diabetic ketoacidosis (DKA)

c. 15-year-old with a broken leg in traction.

b. 80-year-old who had abdominal surgery

d. 60-year-old stroke victim with right-sided paralysis

Answer: C

Remember a "known" patient can develop a new problem

Figure 3.1	*Teaching critical thinking—Critical thinking course content and prioritization handout (cont.)*

Avoid the "Oh my GOD!" distracter (red herring)

Question: A nurse decides to help out when coming upon a head-on collision car accident that just occurred. The nurse notes the victim has bright red blood spurting from the shoulder and a detached arm is lying at the patient's side. The right leg is turned 180 degrees, facing backwards. The nurse should first

    a. apply direct pressure to the source of the spurting blood.

    b. assess for a pedal pulse in the deformed leg.

    c. check for a carotid pulse

    d. verify that the airway is open.

Answer: D

Remember to avoid WHO rather than "what"

Just because someone is more demanding or "ranked" higher should not distract from a more urgent patient need. Express your limit. "I understand you need me. I have to take care of this urgent need first and then I can work with you."

Question: Which of the following should the nurse take care of first?

    a. The bathroom sink has a leak.

    b. An irate family member is in the hall, demanding to see the supervisor.

    c. A patient is lying on the floor, having fallen and hit her head.

    d. A physician is at the nurse's station and wants to discuss an order.

Answer: C

Remember, prioritization does not mean a person's need is not met. It is first things first so the right care is given to the right person at the right time for the right reason.

Source: Polly Gerber Zimmermann, RN, MS, MBA, CEN

Figure	Teaching critical thinking skills—
3.2	Sample course content, objectives, and scenarios

SAMPLE COURSE CONTENT

Sample course objectives

1. Identify four mechanisms or thought processes that are examples of critical thinking.

2. List two validations for the need of accurate baseline assessments.

3. Describe the hospital policy on patient reassessments.

4. Relate an atypical geriatric patient scenario that involves the cardiopulmonary system.

5. Identify two medications commonly prescribed to the geriatric patient that may mask signs/symptoms of shock.

6. Relate two responsibilities of the nurse that require critical thinking skills.

7. Describe the use of pertinent negatives and positives in nursing documentation.

Sample course content

- Patient assessment
  - Reviewing collected data and making a decision
  - Using pertinent negatives and positives
  - Common errors
  - How vital are vital signs?

- Documentation
  - When to document
  - What not to document
  - Where to document

Figure 3.2	Teaching critical thinking skills— Sample course content, objectives, and scenarios (cont.)

- When to call the physician
  - Age-specific concerns

- Red flags of assessment
  - Case scenarios

- Incorporating policy and procedure

- Professional responsibilities
  - Scope of practice
  - Risk management

Sample scenarios for student workbook or discussion

Case 1

Temp 97.4° (rectal)   Pulse 118   Respirations 26   Blood Pressure 128/72

Which vital sign is not only out of the normal range, but of most concern to you?

What are you concerned about with this adult patient?

What should you assess on this patient to determine if there is a potential for demise?

Case 2

Temp 102.4° (oral)   Pulse 78   Respirations 14   Blood Pressure 78/52

In the adult patient, what is of concern to you with these vital signs?

What other information do you need to determine if there is a potential for demise?

Source: Shelley Cohen, RN, BS, CEN

Figure 3.3 — *Teaching critical thinking skills— Classroom tips*

TIPS FOR A SUCCESSFUL CLASS

1. Incorporate anatomy and physiology

- Hand out crayons or colored pencils

- Use applicable anatomy sheets from *www.enchantedlearning.com*

- Display (slide or poster) the anatomy section you want them to fill in

- Identify a specific area (for example, the brain) and have them color it a certain color)

- When completed, display a correct completed anatomy picture and have learners self-correct their drawings

2. Incorporate policy and procedures

- Identify policy/procedure appropriate to case scenarios you are using
- Ask if they know where to retrieve/access the policy/procedure
- Emphasize standards of practice

3. Case scenarios

- Use as many as you can fit into the time period
- If multiple specialty areas are in the class, vary the scenarios
- Relate critical-thinking strategies as you go through the cases

Figure	Teaching critical thinking skills—
3.3	*Classroom tips (cont.)*

4. Documentation

- Use your standard nursing documentation forms or a printout of your electronic form
- Give them a case scenario and have them document the patient assessment
- Go around the room and have a few participants read their charts
- Display a correct documentation note for the patient case
- Discuss risk-management concerns related to documentation

5. Resources

- If you can access the Internet in your classroom setting, search for clinical scenarios that have photos (e.g., a rash, EKG and pose questions to the participants)

- Use tools such as crossword puzzles to help participants improve their prioritizing skills

6. Evaluation

Obtain feedback from participants to determine if they would like a follow-up to this critical thinking–skills course. Give them course content options and let them check off which they are interested in:

- More anatomy and physiology
- Laboratory results
- IV fluids
- Critical situation scenarios
- Interventions for an emergency

7. Self assessment tools

Incorporate a self-assessment tool that participants can complete and use to work with preceptors or managers (Figure 3.4). Consider having them complete the same form before and after the class to validate the need for the course and to show them how attending has improved their critical thinking skills.

Source: Shelley Cohen, RN, BS, CEN

Figure 3.4	Teaching critical thinking skills— Sample self-assessment tool

CRITICAL THINKING SELF-ASSESSMENT

Use the following scale to respond to each statement:

4 = I feel very comfortable with this

3 = I feel somewhat comfortable with this

2 = I feel somewhat uncomfortable with this

1 = I feel very uncomfortable with this

1.	Calling the physician at 3 a.m. regarding a patient's status	4	3	2	1
2.	Identifying a patient at risk for an immediate demise	4	3	2	1
3.	Initiating emergency measures until help arrives	4	3	2	1
4.	Relating changes in vital signs to the individual patient scenario	4	3	2	1
5.	Knowing when to bring a patient-care concern to the attention of the charge nurse / team leader	4	3	2	1
6.	Identifying age-specific red flags that would alert me to reassess the patient	4	3	2	1
7.	Knowing what to document and what not to document	4	3	2	1
8.	Identifying patient situations that may be a risk for myself or the organization	4	3	2	1
9.	Verbally relaying to another professional my concerns regarding a patient's status	4	3	2	1

Source: Shelley Cohen, RN, BS, CEN

Figure 3.5   *Teaching critical thinking skills—Handout*

Sample pocket card. Print out, fold in half, laminate (if possible), and give to attendees of the critical thinking class.

Attributes of a critical thinker

- Asks pertinent questions
- Assesses statements and arguments
- Is curious about things
- Listens to others and is able to give feedback
- Looks for evidence or proof
- Examines problems closely
- Can reject information that is not relevant or is incorrect
- Wants to find the solution
- Thinks independently
- Questions deeply
- Has intellectual integrity
- Is confident in rationale for actions
- Analyzes arguments
- Evaluates evidence and facts
- Explores consequences before taking action
- Recognizes a contradiction
- Evaluates policy

When to call the provider

- Perfusion problem
- Pain issue
- Standing-order concern
- Atypical presentation complaints
- Risk-management potential
- What's going in isn't coming out
- Negative response to intervention
- Social concerns / family issues affecting patient care

Reference: Ferrett, S. 1997. *Peak Performance: Success in College and Beyond.* New York: McGraw-Hill.

Source: Shelley Cohen, RN, BS, CEN

Orientation: Bringing critical thinking to the clinical environment

LEARNING OBJECTIVES

After reading this section, the participant should be able to

- determine ways to evaluate nurses' progress in critical thinking throughout orientation
- develop strategies for the development of critical thinking skills during the orientation process

Moving from the classroom to the bedside

As educators and nurse leaders start to think about developing a process to move teaching critical thinking from the classroom to the work setting, consider these questions:

- Can nurses who learn critical thinking in the classroom setting apply it in the clinical environment?

- How do you evaluate their ability to apply this knowledge?

- Does your orientation process incorporate critical thinking and how you do a baseline assessment on the new staff you hire?

- Are experienced nursing staff given the education they need so they may learn to identify key opportunities to develop critical thinking in your new staff?

If you focus on critical thinking from the beginning of orientation through to the annual review process, nurses will understand the vital role it plays in delivering safe patient care. Incorporating critical thinking into ongoing orientation processes allows you to build a nursing culture that embraces the concept of critical thinking from the date of hire.

Beginning with orientation

When you mention orientation to a new nursing staff members they typically think of sitting in a classroom to learn specifics about your organization. They expect you to address medication policies, fire safety, and the Joint Commission on Accreditation of Healthcare Organizations (JCAHO), among other regulatory requirements. They also expect to take a medication test to validate that they can apply their skills in the clinical arena.

Since nurses know these items will be addressed as part of the orientation process, this is an ideal setting to introduce your expectations on critical thinking abilities, both for new graduate nurses and for those with more experience.

Self-assessment

Once orientees have undergone classroom education regarding critical thinking, they will naturally conduct their own internal review of the information to figure out how well they function with the concepts. It is to be expected that new graduate nurses will demonstrate the most hesitancy in this area.

Regardless of the years of experience of your new hires, conducting a self assessment is a valuable tool to measure their perception of their ability to perform at the critical-thinking level. Figure 4.1, on page 55, is an example of a tool that can be used to measure nurses' critical thinking skills for general nursing responsibilities. Figure 4.2, on page 57, is tailored for OB-specific skills during the OB part of orientation. Give either or both of these forms to new hires to complete at the start of orientation. The forms should be reviewed by the new hires and by their preceptors, and occasionally even their managers.

| Figure 4.1 | *Critical thinking self-assessment tool—General nursing skills* |

Employee name: _____

Date of hire: _____

Position hired for: _____

This self-assessment tool will help guide your preceptor and manager throughout your orientation process to ensure we provide you with the tools and resources you need for success.

How comfortable are you at doing the things listed below?

	I feel very comfortable with this	I feel somewhat comfortable with this	I feel somewhat uncomfortable with this	I feel very uncomfortable with this	Comments
Calling the doctor at 3:00 a.m. about a patient's status					
Identifying a patient at risk for immediate demise					
Initiating emergency measures until help arrives					
Identifying possible causes of vital sign changes related to the patient's condition					

	Figure
4.1	***Critical thinking self-assessment tool—***
	General nursing skills (cont.)

	I feel very comfortable with this	I feel somewhat comfortable with this	I feel somewhat uncomfortable with this	I feel very uncomfortable with this	Comments
Knowing when to bring a patient-care concern to the attention of the charge nurse					
Identifying age-specific alerts that indicate the patient needs reevaluation					
Knowing what to document and what not to document					
Identifying patient scenarios that may be a risk-management concern					
Verbally relaying concerns to another professional					

Source: Shelley Cohen, RN, BS, CEN

Figure 4.2	*Critical thinking self-assessment tool—Pediatric nursing skills*

Employee name: _____

Date of hire: _____

Position hired for: _____

This self-assessment tool will help guide your preceptor and manager throughout your orientation process to ensure we provide you with the tools and resources you need for success.

How comfortable are you at doing the things listed below?

	I feel very comfortable with this	I feel somewhat comfortable with this	I feel somewhat uncomfortable with this	I feel very uncomfortable with this	Comments
Identifying red flags that an infant is dehydrated					
Defining my role when a patient has a critical lab value					
Making a decision during the assessment process that reflects the seriousness of the child's presentation					
Anticipating needs of patients presenting with commonly seen pediatric emergencies					

| | Figure 4.2 | Critical thinking self-assessment tool—Pediatric nursing skills (cont.) |

	I feel very comfortable with this	I feel somewhat comfortable with this	I feel somewhat uncomfortable with this	I feel very uncomfortable with this	Comments
Identifying verbal and nonverbal clues that my patient may be a victim of abuse or neglect					
Recognizing signals that a parent or visitor has the potential for violent behavior					
Redirecting the pediatrician to the patient in greatest need of intervention					
Providing age-appropriate preparation for the preschool child prior to treatments and procedures					
Preparing the parents for providing care to their child at home					
Providing privacy and respecting adolescents' developmental needs					

Source: Shelley Cohen, RN, BS, CEN and June Marshall, RN, MS, CNAA,BC

©2007 HCPro, Inc.
Critical Thinking in the Pediatric Unit

When developing your own self-assessment tool, or adapting the ones included, make sure to include items that reflect

- generic nursing skill
- specialty-area questions
- questions for both the novice and experienced nurse

New hires should be asked to complete the same self-assessment tools when they conclude their orientation period, or after about three months. You can then compare the responses to the initial assessment, which also could be reviewed by the preceptor and/or manager. Keep in mind that the responses may show no difference when the experience or knowledge level of nurses is at its peak performance level. Others should show marked improvements during this period, particularly new graduate nurses.

Having new employees conduct a self-assessment at the beginning of orientation and again after they have been at your facility for a few months helps by

- clarifying and defining their critical thinking abilities and identifying areas that require more attention during orientation

- providing a documentation process that validates areas of strength and weakness

- becoming a resource tool from which you and the nurse may develop goals

- providing a record of the dates that orientees demonstrated these proficiencies

The role of preceptors

As new hires transition through the orientation process, their assigned preceptors will be key to the application of critical thinking in the clinical practice area. Regardless of experience level, new hires will look to their preceptors as role models for critical thinking skills.

Before preceptors can teach critical thinking to orientees, they must first be practicing the skills themselves. Therefore, make sure you pick clinically competent critical thinkers who will be suitable role models for the type of nursing care you want practiced. It is also important that the organization invest time and education in training preceptors so they can meet your expectations.

Preceptors should be provided with guidelines and goals to follow as they orient new employees. This will help them to

- validate successful goals in the new hire

- clearly identify areas that require remediation

- present organized documentation to show that the new hire is able to meet the requirements of the job for which they were hired

New hires who quickly display critical thinking skills will bring a great sense of relief to their preceptors. All new hires should display skills as they progress through their development, but those who show evidence earlier than others take quite a load off the mind of the preceptor.

How can preceptors teach critical thinking?

Preceptors can help orientees develop and stimulate the use of critical thinking skills by following some of these suggestions.

Minimizing the emphasis on ability to perform skills and tasks: New hires are eager to complete the required "check-offs" for competencies related to performing clinical tasks. Preceptors should encourage them to focus on other aspects of their orientation as well, for example, finding the facility's policy on dealing with patients who want to leave AMA.

Maximizing emphasis on the ability to recognize when the skill or task is needed: As new hires request to be "checked off" on various skills or tasks, preceptors should ask questions to demonstrate whether new hires have the ability to critically think through why the patient needs this particular task or skill performed.

Encourage a realistic time frame and expectations: Display time-related goals for the new hire so the peer group will not have unrealistic expectations of when the new hire will be comfortable with something. Post a spreadsheet that lists the names of the orientees and goals for the next 30 days. Affix dates to the items so preceptors may check them off when successfully completed. This serves to keep all staff up to date on what orientees are competent to do, and ensures they do not delegate a task for which an orientee is not yet prepared. It also keeps a check on any unrealistic expectations staff nurses may have for new hires. Staff nurses can look at the list and know that orientees cannot admit a patient on their own because that skill will not be taught until the next time sheet.

Do not assume the new hire understands the what, why, how, or when of delivering nursing care: If the orientee is a seasoned nurse, the preceptor should not make assumptions that length of experience is directly related to knowledge and ability to use critical thinking skills. Instead, all new hires should be required to demonstrate the same knowledge. The preceptor can use prompting questions to begin the what, why, how, and when questioning to allow the new hire to demonstrate appropriate reasoning.

Figure 4.3 serves as a helpful guide for both the preceptor and the orientee to validate this process of finding out the what, why, how, and when.

Figure 4.3	Preceptor tool—Relating skills to critical thinking for new graduate nurses

RELATING SKILLS TO CRITICAL THINKING

	Why does my patient need this?	How will I know if it is working?	What else should I consider/observe?	How long will my patient need it for?
Central venous access for intravenous therapy				
Oxygen therapy				
Cardiac/apnea monitor				
Septic work-up				
Nasogastric tube feeding				
Pain assessment and management				
Foley catheter				
Referral to Child Protective Services				
Chest physiotherapy				
Chest tube with suction				
Enteric precautions				

Source: Shelley Cohen, RN, BS, CEN and June Marshall, RN, MS, CNAA,BC

 ©2007 HCPro, Inc.   **Critical Thinking in the Pediatric Unit**

Teachable moments

Once new hires are in the clinical setting, there are numerous opportunities for the preceptor to teach and demonstrate the application of critical thinking with actual patients. This is also the time when new hires to reveal their ability to apply the knowledge they started learning in the orientation classroom.

Examples of "teachable moments" include

- preparation of assignment/organization during their shift

- information shared during shift report

- early identification of patients in need of specific interventions that can involve new hires

- prompting the what/why/how/when questions for specific patient scenarios

Figure 4.4 is a tool to encourage the critical thinking of the orientee, and can be filled in to provide further examples of situations that present teachable moments. Adapt the problem list in this figure to include items directly related to your clinical practice area.

Figure 4.4			Preceptor tool—Relating patient observations to critical thinking		

DEALING WITH PROBLEMS OR SITUATIONS

Problem or situation	What does the patient need?	Why does the patient need this?	How do I do this?	When should I do this?	What should I document? Where do I document?
Postoperative day three and the child's abdominal wound is red, warm, and painful					
The 2-year-old patient is wheezing and having in-creased work of breathing					
The mother of a 9-month-old child admitted with a skull fracture shows no signs of concern or sad-ness about the child's injury					

 ©2007 HCPro, Inc.   **Critical Thinking in the Pediatric Unit**

Figure 4.4			**Preceptor tool—Relating patient observations to critical thinking (cont.)**		

Problem or situation	What does the patient need?	Why does the patient need this?	How do I do this?	When should I do this?	What should I document? Where do I document?
The provider orders a dose of acetamino-phen for an infant that exceeds the recommenda-tions for the child's weight and age					
The 14-year-old patient is found gagging herself and vomiting in the bathroom after her meals					

Source: Shelley Cohen, RN, BS, CEN and June Marshall, RN, MS, CNAA,BC

Sometimes nursing staff other than the preceptor may be working with the orientee. During these times, it is essential that the preceptor educate all staff on the importance of their role in assisting with the transition process of the newly hired nurse.

The preceptor can promote and encourage positive behaviors among staff that will help to promote and motivate the critical thinking process. Figure 4.5 is a tool preceptors can share with other staff to encourage their understanding and support for developing new employees' critical thinking. It has essential reminders that include

- faster is not always clinically better

- checking things off for a new hire indicates you observed them perform it

- proactively involve new hires in challenging patient scenarios—but be there to support them

- ask prompting questions that validate they can apply knowledge

- knowing where your department resources are is as important as learning tasks and skills

Figure 4.5	***Preceptor tool—Promote and support critical thinking***

EVERYONE CAN PROMOTE AND SUPPORT CRITICAL THINKING

To encourage newly hired nurses in their orientation process, we all need to provide a supportive and nurturing clinical environment. We want team members who can answer the what/why/how/when of nursing process.

Here's how you can help to create this environment.

1. **Faster is not necessarily better, as long as it's done correctly**

   Does it really matter—in many situations—if it takes new hires a few minutes longer to get in the IV? Yes, you could have done it faster—but how fast did you do it when you were a new nurse?

2. **Make no assumptions about skills**

   If you are asked to check off a new hire on a skill, be sure you actually observe the performance of this skill and then ask:

   - Why does/did this patient need a _____?
   - How did you know the correct way to perform this?
   - Where did you find the information?
   - How will you tell if the procedure is helpful for the patient?
   - What and where will you document what you have done?

3. **When you identify a challenging patient scenario or a procedure not commonly performed, invite the new hire to participate**

   This will help increase the experience of the new hire, as well as help the team identify the new hire's willingness to learn.

| Figure 4.5 | Preceptor tool—Promote and support critical thinking (cont.) |

4. **At shift change report ask prompting questions in a non-defensive manner**

    - What do you think is going on with this patient?
    - Are you comfortable with what the provider told you after you spoke with him or her?

5. **Observe new hires' ability to prioritize and organize their assignments**

    - Is there a particular reason you have not done the pre-op teaching yet on Mrs. Jones?

    - You look concerned. Is everything ok? Let's go over your assignment and talk about priorities for the shift. I'd like to hear what you think are the most important issues in these patients and why.

6. **When questions arise, do they know where to look for the answers or are they simply expecting coworkers to answer them?**

    - I am not sure about these medicines being compatible. How could you find out?

    - When you are not sure whether a permit is needed for a procedure, where could you find that information?

Source: Shelley Cohen, RN, BS, CEN

Evaluating skills

As new nurses work their way through the orientation process, evaluating their ability to apply critical thinking in their clinical setting needs to be accomplished. Sometimes knowing what to do is as important as knowing what not to do. The preceptor needs evidence of new hires' abilities to assess the needs of each patient.

The following should be assessed:

- Evaluate a patient's health status: Are their patient assessment skills targeted to the patient's presentation?

- Identify potential scenarios based on the patient's health status: Are they aware of potential problems or complications this patient may be at risk for?

- Evaluate a patient's response to interventions: Are they performing an appropriate reassessment? Can they identify if the patient is the same, worse, or better?

- Evaluate the need for higher skill level: If patient is not responding to intervention, do they know what to do next?

- Take action when indicated: Can they initiate actions needed by patients, such as standing orders? Are they able to prioritize these actions?

Handling judgment or action errors during orientation

In any moment of decision the best thing to do is the right thing, the next best thing is the wrong thing, and the worst thing you can do is nothing.

—Theodore Roosevelt

It is more encouraging to see an orientee taking action in the clinical setting than those who elect to do nothing about a patient situation. The fact that they are willing to do something shows they are making progress. And the reality is that an error of judgment may be made by an experienced nurse as well as a new graduate.

It's important to understand that placing an experienced nurse in a new and unfamiliar clinical specialty area creates an opportunity for judgment or action errors, just as new graduates may make errors due to their unfamiliarity with nursing. Experienced nurses who have moved to a new clinical specialty will be exposed to unfamiliar medications, procedures, and age-specific considerations. For example, an experienced emergency nurse who transitions to the pediatric unit is going into a world of very different patients. The nurse's medication dosing was very different for adults in the emergency setting than it will be for pediatric patients. In addition, he or she will experience different situations and interactions with patients. For the most part, he or she did not develop relationships with ED patients for more than a few hours and may never have met patients' families for any additional medical information. Now, the nurse will have to interact with stressed and anxious parents, while caring for sick children.

Accept that errors will occur and lay the groundwork for making sure errors are handled in the correct manner. Preceptors and the entire peer group play a large role in the recovery process when errors occur, and should help ensure that incidents become an opportunity to develop critical thinking skills that will reduce such incidents in the future.

In addition, the response of the preceptor and peers to these scenarios will determine whether new hires feel supported during what is a challenging time for them. Nurses are often quick to "quarterback" incidents with comments about how "We would never have done that" or "I would never have done that first." Remember that orientation is a time of learning, setting goals, and identifying areas of strength and weakness. Newly hired nurses should not be left with a feeling of "being chewed up and spit out" by their peer group.

All incidents can be used as learning experiences. When errors occur, they may reveal some positive attributes about the new hire:

- The nurse was willing to be held accountable and identified the error to you

- The nurse was grateful and appreciative that you pointed out the error

- The nurse requested resources for self-learning to better understand the red flags that he or she missed with the patient

- The nurse asked questions to better understand how the patient got to this point

- The nurse sought guidance in completing a reporting form if one was needed

Preceptors or mentors of new employees must identify the decisions that were or were not made by the nurse that reflect a lack of critical thinking. Once these are recognized, then the preceptor can become the teacher to guide the nurse as he or she learns so that a similar situation is not replayed in the future.

Remediation

Working with new hires on remediation after an event is a delicate job. How you handle the situation will greatly affect how much they learn, how they feel and whether they can accept what happened, and whether they develop their critical thinking skills so as to understand the situation.

These teaching qualities will help you have a successful interaction:

Patience: What is obvious critical thinking to you may not be for others. You may need to provide repetition in the learning process and allow time for the nurse to digest the information before requiring him or her to demonstrate understanding.

Support: Being supportive after an error in judgment does not mean you minimize the importance of what occurred. It simply reflects that you support the nurse. Some words to use to send a supportive and reassuring message include

- I understand you are upset about what happened with Mr. Smith

- I realize this material is all new to you—let's go over it again

- Take a step back and look at all the things you have accomplished

- Good for you for recognizing and notifying me of the error—it takes courage and strong ethics to do so

Clarification: Define in writing for the new hire what you expect of him or her in light of what has occurred. If you discussed timelines, include those in the written expectations. For the new hire who simply does not have the capacity to apply critical thinking, it is essential that your documentation reflect what happened, what steps were taken, and what improvements were expected to occur so as to validate any future employment decisions. Examples of written expectations include

- all medication doses requiring calculations will be reviewed with the preceptor prior to administering to the patient.

- there will be no further incidents of patients signing out AMA without nursing documentation that "tells the story" of these events. The orientee will develop a list of other risk-management scenarios related to the department and present these at our next scheduled orientation meeting.

Realism: Keep in mind the reality of the situation. It is not about what you learned in nursing school or when you went through orientation years ago. It is about the present situation and the circumstances and experiences of the new nurse.

- Remember that not all new grads are clinically prepared at the same level

- Review critical thinking goals and timelines to ensure they are appropriate

- Recognize those nurses who may never be able to meet these goals successfully, and deal with the situation appropriately

Orientation sets critical-thinking expectations

The orientation process and critical thinking should go hand in hand. Orientation allows new hires to see how the critical thinking skills they learned in the classroom can be integrated into practice. It is the foundation upon which they can build on their development from novice to expert.

 ©2007 HCPro, Inc.   **Critical Thinking in the Pediatric Unit**

Figure
4.6

Successful orientation requires critical thinking

Successful critical thinking starts at the point of hire with the orientation process. It takes the entire team and each of these components to develop critical thinking.

Assess current critical thinking skills related to assigned specialty area

Assess current critical thinking skills related to general nursing principles

Successful orientation is tied to critical thinking

Educate clinical staff on how to assess and develop critical thinking

Reassess during clinical orientation and reevaluate ability to apply critical thinking skills

Source: Shelley Cohen, RN, BS, CEN

Nursing practice that promotes and motivates critical thinking

---

LEARNING OBJECTIVE

After reading this section, the participant should be able to

- discuss the role played by managers and educators in promoting environments that support critical thinking

Maintaining momentum

Once nurses have finished with orientation, the journey to critical thinking becomes more subtle.

After spending time and money to teach nursing staff about critical thinking skills, you probably have high hopes for seeing these skills translated into improvements in patient care. Yet if you do not create an environment that supports and motivates ongoing development of critical thinking, it is unrealistic to expect most staff to continue to practice it.

Immediately after completing a course on critical thinking, most experienced nurses will independently implement critical thinking in their daily practice. But without a setting that supports the ongoing development and use of these skills, nurses will easily fall back into practice patterns that do not involve a higher level of reasoning. New graduate nurses have no previous experiences or practices to fall back on, but the reality of practice may reduce their ability to think critically. How they are mentored and the role models of experienced nurses around them will determine what they will offer for patient care.

Nurses respond well to challenging work environments and practice settings that embrace critical thinking. Nurses who practice critical thinking operate at a higher level, meaning they are more likely to be stimulated and fulfilled professionally. This may be demonstrated by

- interest in committee involvement
- support for quality improvement efforts
- proactively seeking to attend ongoing education
- initiating more collaborate efforts with other members of the team
- early identification of acute changes in patients

In addition to the preceptor/mentor, the following people and practices play important roles in encouraging the ongoing development and implementation of critical thinking and practice standards. Identify the areas in which you can implement the most immediate change.

- Nurse manager

- Nurse educator

- Defining critical-thinking expectations in a written format through
  - job descriptions
  - clinical guidelines
  - policy and procedure

Nurse managers and staff educators

Newly hired and seasoned staff will look to nurse managers, as the leader of the department(s), to validate how much importance they should place on this "critical thinking stuff." They will look to staff educators to provide leadership and ongoing education.

Nurse managers and staff educators should set expectations for critical thinking by expecting staff to have the ability to

- organize
- prioritize
- delegate
- practice safely
- apply reasoning when making decisions

These are the skills of nurses who have the ability to make appropriate decisions, and they will have been discussed through classroom sessions and during orientation. But if managers and educators do not maintain the momentum through a culture that requires ongoing development of critical thinking, your orientation efforts will fall short. You need to ensure a patient-care environment that nurtures critical thinkers, that stimulates them and motivates them to engage in a discussion in their minds. This discussion is all about one question: *Is this in the best interest of the patient?*

Take out one of your time sheets, and as you look down the list of names, ask yourself how you really feel about each nurse's ability to demonstrate these attributes. Use Figure 5.1 to assist you as you validate educational and remediation needs of individual staff. This tool also may be used by preceptors and senior staff—such as charge nurses—who are involved in assessing staff performance.

Figure

5.1

Critical thinking skills assessment—
Nurse manager/staff educator tool

Staff name	1	2	3	4	5	6	7	8	9	10	11	12	13	14	15

1. Asks pertinent questions
2. Assesses statements/arguments
3. Displays curiosity
4. Listens to others and gives feedback
5. Looks for evidence or proof
6. Examines problems closely
7. Rejects incorrect information
8. Wants to find answers
9. Independently thinks things through
10. Displays confidence about actions
11. Can analyze an argument
12. Looks at the evidence and facts
13. Considers consequences before acting
14. Recognizes contradictions
15. Evaluates policy and considers appropriateness for patient

Source: Shelley Cohen, RN, BS, CEN

Making critical thinking part of the culture

For critical thinking to be a part of your nursing culture, it has to be more than something that is simply "checked off" once a year. The concepts of reasoning should be ingrained in the following:

- job descriptions
- clinical guidelines
- policy and procedure
- performance reviews
- processes that incorporate goal setting

Job descriptions

Job descriptions that do not reflect the reality of what staff members actually do or are expected to do provide no foundation for staff accountability, but it is impossible to include every item, task, or responsibility that nurses will be expected to perform. Therefore, using terminology related to critical thinking sends a clear message that "other duties" may be required.

To improve the content of your job descriptions, consider

- Involving staff in the process of updating and reviewing job descriptions on a regular basis. Ask prompting questions to assist staff in this process:

  - What are you doing on a regular basis that is not on the job description?
  - What is on the job description that you no longer do?
  - What do you feel should be added that will help hold all nurses more accountable?

- Identify patient scenarios that demonstrated a lack of critical thinking:

  - Was there anything absent from the job description that made it difficult to hold staff accountable for their action or lack of action?

- Were there practice standards related to the scenario that were not followed? If so, do the current job descriptions define the expectation that staff members are responsible for maintaining a current knowledge base for the specialty in which they provide nursing care?

Job description examples

- Nurses will use critical thinking skills to determine action needed for risk management concerns such as medical restraint of patients; adolescent patient elopement; violent or combative patient, visitor, or family behavior; and suspected child abuse or neglect.

- The reassessment process for children who are medically immobilized/restrained is dictated by policy, but nurses are expected to critically think through the specific needs of each patient and understand which patients may require more frequent monitoring than policy dictates.

- Pediatric nurses will use critical thinking skills when determining the impact of the patient's growth and developmental level upon the presenting disease or condition and vice versa.

- Pediatric nurses will use critical thinking skills to manage their workload and offer support to other team members as indicated by patient acuity and staff skill mix on the unit.

Clinical guidelines

We all know staff members who attend training events and seminars, yet do not have the ability to apply what they learned in the clinical setting. An example of this may be the nurse who successfully passes the PALS written exam and the testing stations, yet he or she is disorganized and lacks knowledge in an actual resuscitative event. The same principle applies to critical thinking concepts. The nurse may have been taught critical thinking principles, yet when performing patient care he or she does not appear to "have it together." This may present itself as disorganization or even in an actual patient error from a lack of judgment.

Clinical guidelines—also referred to as care paths and clinical pathways—provide evidence-based interventions and direction to set standards of practice for specific patient clinical presentations.

These models require the nurse to use reasoning and prioritization to determine when to take each step in the guideline. (If nurses are unable to follow clinical guidelines, they need remediation and further help.)

The implementation of clinical guidelines demonstrates the use of standards of practice, as well as implying that nurses possess the critical thinking needed to apply the guidelines.

Policy and procedure

When relating policy and procedure to critical thinking, you should expect nurses to grasp the following:

- Know where policies and procedures are kept
- Read the policies and procedures
- Understand what each policy is asking/requiring
- Identify the patient/situation for which to engage each policy or procedure

---

Policy and procedure examples

Reassessment of the pediatric patient

The pediatric nurse will use critical thinking skills in determining what physiologic and psychosocial aspects of the patient's presenting condition require reassessment, how frequently the reassessment should occur, and how the findings should best be communicated and documented.

Pediatric visitation policies

The pediatric nurse will employ critical thinking to identify those situations that may require exceptions to standard visitation policies. In a family-centered care environment, parents are not considered visitors and should be permitted to stay with their child at all times. Visitation may cause difficulty for staff when divorced parents have custody battles, and visitation decisions regarding extended family members, step parents, or spouses' significant others may produce conflict between the parents. Peer visitation for adolescents can also become problematic in some situations and must be handled carefully by the nurse to protect adolescent's rights, while maintaining a safe environment.

Figure **5.2**			***Annual performance review— Self-assessment of critical thinking***			

Employee name: _____ **Date of self-assessment:** _____

Please rate your ability to apply critical thinking in the following areas:

    5 = I always do this

    4 = I do this most of the time

    3 = I sometimes do this

    2 = I rarely do this and realize I need to be more aware in this area

    1 = I never do this and realize I need some help to improve on this

1.	I ask pertinent questions.	5	4	3	2	1
2.	I assess statements/arguments before making decisions.	5	4	3	2	1
3.	I am always curious about things and want to learn.	5	4	3	2	1
4.	I listen to others and give feedback.	5	4	3	2	1
5.	I look for evidence or proof before doing what someone else says I should do.	5	4	3	2	1
6.	I examine problems closely.	5	4	3	2	1
7.	I know when information is incorrect and I reject it.	5	4	3	2	1
8.	I want to find answers.	5	4	3	2	1
9.	I independently think things through.	5	4	3	2	1
10.	I am confident in my actions.	5	4	3	2	1
11.	I can analyze an argument..	5	4	3	2	1
12.	I look at the evidence and facts.	5	4	3	2	1
13.	I consider consequences before acting.	5	4	3	2	1
14.	I recognize contradictions.	5	4	3	2	1
15.	I evaluate policy and consider its appropriateness for the patient.	5	4	3	2	1

Source: Shelley Cohen, RN, BS, CEN

©2007 HCPro, Inc.
Critical Thinking in the Pediatric Unit

Performance reviews

The annual review is an opportunity for the manager to reinforce expectations regarding critical thinking with each member of the nursing staff. Again, Figure 5.1 (page 78) can be used or adapted to outline areas of strength and weakness for each nurse. You also may want to have the nursing staff perform a self-assessment of their ability to think critically prior to the annual review. Figure 5.2 is an example of a self-assessment tool.

This self-assessment tool can be compared to the worksheet you prepared for the employee's performance review and the employee's goals for the coming year (Figure 5.3 can be used to plan short- and long-term goals), and can be specific to discuss judgment and reasoning when appropriate. Other benefits of staff performing a self-assessment of their abilities are

- it details specific expectations from both you and the patient

- in the process of completing the tool, questions should and will arise regarding critical-thinking concepts, prompting further discussion

- it requires them to consider specific patient scenarios when they have actually displayed these abilities

Figure	Goals worksheet
5.3	

Name: _____

Job title: _____

Today's date: _____

Short-term goals

In the next year, I would like to do the following:

Add _____ to my job description

Take _____ continuing education classes

Work on projects related to improving _____

Long-term goals

In the next 2–5 years I would like to do the following:

Have completed _____

Make these changes in my job _____

Have accomplished _____

Obtain certification in _____

Source: Shelley Cohen, RN, BS, CEN

 ©2007 HCPro, Inc.   **Critical Thinking in the Pediatric Unit**

As you and the nurse identify areas that need improvement, first prompt the nurse to offer suggestions and resources before you do. Remember, part of your role is to coach staff—if you provide all the answers all the time, you are stifling their critical thinking.

Goal setting

When staff demonstrate unacceptable behavior or unsafe patient practices, take the opportunity to discuss the importance of critical thinking. From point of hire to annual review to daily patient care, judgment will always play a central role. When setting new goals in response to unacceptable behavior or unsafe patient events, relate the goals to the nurse developing better judgment and displaying higher levels of critical thinking.

Figure 5.4 contains examples of what to consider saying and how to document the conversation and conclusions reached.

Figure 5.4	Setting goals for improvement

Should Nancy present to the department late on another shift between today's date and _____ she will know that

- an off-going shift member will be delayed
- an oncoming shift nurse will have to take an additional assignment
- patient care will be directly affected

Nancy has the ability to critically think through the ramifications for when staff do not present on time for their shift and she has outlined these in our meeting today.

Timothy is aware of the resources available to nurses in the department when they are in need of detailed medication information. He agrees that if he had looked up the information on _____ and applied nursing judgment, the patient would not have been given the dose.

Timothy will demonstrate appropriate nursing judgment when administering medication by

- using available resources in the department such as reference books by or calling the pharmacy.

- successfully completing a written medication assessment tool, achieving a grade of 90% or better. This will be done within the next 15 days.

- having the charge nurse check all calculations for pediatric medications for the next 30 days.

Source: Shelley Cohen, RN, BS, CEN

Novice to expert: Setting realistic expectations for critical thinking

LEARNING OBJECTIVES

After reading this section, the participant should be able to

- analyze the challenges that both new and experienced nurses face in the incorporation of critical thinking skills in the practice setting
- explain interventions to help both new and experienced nurses meet their managers and preceptors expectations for critical thinking

Setting realistic expectations

As you approach and consider methods not only to teach but also to motivate critical thinking, it is essential that your expectations meet the abilities of the nurse. The last thing you want is an environment that creates fear of critical-thinking expectations. We want staff to embrace the concept, confident in their abilities to develop their thinking and reasoning skills.

Align your expectations more with what it is realistic to expect from nurses, rather than what you hope they can do. As you set your expectations, consider each nurse's potential, opportunities to perform, opportunities to reach goals, and the outcomes you hope each nurse will achieve.

Make sure your expectations are

- realistic
- supported with appropriate tools and resources
- appropriate for the specialty area in which the nurse works
- flexible to meet a variety of learning needs
- clarified in writing
- related to the performance review

Novice to competent: New graduate nurses

It may seem obvious that the expectations for critical thinking displayed by new graduate nurses would not be the same as those for experienced nurses. Yet many new graduate nurses are facing peer groups who have already decided what they should/should not know. Preceptors, nurse educators, and nurse managers are the ones who must set the expectations for new graduates, not the experienced nurses on the unit. Preceptors, nurse educators, and nurse managers should be the ones who communicate the expectations for new graduates to the rest of the staff.

When new graduate nurses join the obstetrics unit, use the opportunity for the team to consider the experience of new nurses and what new graduates have to cope with. Include the following points in the discussion to enlighten staff and help them have a better understanding of why the expectations on new graduates are different today than they were in previous decades:

- Many students today have fewer clinical opportunities than most current nurses had in school.

- Students today have to contend with a chronic shortage of nursing faculty across the country.

- Many nursing schools "teach to the boards" and great focus is placed on successful completion of the NCLEX.

- Students' limited clinical time may not have exposed them to challenging patients similar to those seen in your environment.

- In years past, nurses gained several years of experience before becoming specialty nurses. Now many enter a specialty straight out of school.

Let it be known that you will not tolerate staff members who are unwilling to accept today's realities for new graduates. Do not allow statements such as, "Back in my day we were expected to . . . " The manager, preceptor, and educator need to promptly address individuals who make such comments so the message is clear: This is unacceptable behavior. Work together to script appropriate responses that hold those individuals accountable, such as, "We are not practicing 1962 nursing care here. Are you?"

As new graduates move further along and out of their orientation period, assist in the transition from novice staff nurse to competent staff nurse by considering the following:

- Use tools that allow new graduates to self-assess their level of critical thinking

- Reevaluate decision-making skills throughout the orientation process

- Promptly clarify all questions regarding expectations

- Promote a culture and environment that encourage critical thinking

- Remember that critical thinking is a process that develops and grows throughout the career

- Bear in mind that new graduates who do not employ critical thinking in their personal lives will face the greatest challenges in incorporating it into their nursing care

Greatest challenges for new graduate nurses

Among the many challenges new graduates will face—and obstacles to the development of their critical thinking—are the patients in their care who have bad outcomes and the providers who are unwilling to collaborate with them. The first makes them ask the question, "What should I have done?" The second makes them unwilling to use their critical thinking skills, because they feel they are not needed.

The first year after graduation is a time for education, and care must be taken that new graduates are not frightened to make a decision or feel constantly indecisive in the care they provide.

Coaching new graduates through bad patient outcomes

• Allow them to grieve through their error or omission. Whether patients are in their care for one hour or one week, in their minds, they are still "my patient."

• As nurses we tend to beat ourselves up when we make a medication or other error. After we are done whipping ourselves, we move on. New graduate nurses need time to go through a process where they review what happened and how they would approach it differently next time. Our job is to coach them away from the blame and move them toward learning experiences.

• Provide them with more than one opportunity to sit with a supportive mentor or preceptor to review the scenario that led to the patient outcome.

• Make sure you are the person who debriefs the nurses. Don't expose them to the nurse who says, "I told you this would happen if you let new grads in here."

• Even if the bad outcome was not related to something they did or did not do, they still may feel like it was their fault. Coach them that a guilt trip will not change the outcome of the scenario.

- If they are not willing to take responsibility or accountability for something they did or did not do for the patient, recognize this as a patient safety warning. These nurses will require further assessment of their critical-thinking capabilities and ongoing involvement with the nurse manager.

Growing collaborative relationships with the medical staff

Working with the medical staff can be intimidating for new graduates if steps are not taken to develop relationships. Simple steps can help promote the new relationship and build a basis of good feeling so that both sides may build trust.

- Have someone introduce new graduates to the medical staff as they arrive on the unit.

- If medical staff members have had previous negative experiences with new graduate nurses, make time to discuss the critical-thinking training you are providing these new graduates.

- Circulate a memo to the medical staff introducing the new graduates and briefly outlining expectations, the critical thinking training, and names of the preceptors.

- Ask the members of the medical staff to think back to their own internships and remind them that critical thinking will develop with their support.

- If the new graduates are in a specialty area, see if they can spend some shifts in the offices of those specialties where they can observe and work alongside the practitioner.

- In your critical-thinking training, include scenarios that allow novice nurses to explore options for how to respond to challenging times and conversations with providers. This is part of teaching them how to respond professionally to any challenge in the healthcare environment.

Growing collaborative relationships with the interdisciplinary team

New graduates also face expectations from other team members, which may include ancillary services such as radiology, respiratory therapy, laboratory, and pharmacy. Build a pattern of success for new graduates nurse by communicating with other services:

- Dates of new graduates' arrivals and the departments/areas to which they are assigned

- Include time for new nurses to partner with other services

- Discuss the time frame of the orientation process and give a list of realistic expectations related to their services

- Incorporate interdisciplinary team members' skills and experiences as part of the new graduate's education by including them as faculty for classroom time

When new graduates fail to reach competent levels of critical thinking

For managers and preceptors, one of the greatest challenges is when you are confronted with newly graduated nurses who just don't seem to "get it." There will be times, despite your best efforts and resources, when the concept of critical thinking will not be grasped in a realistic time frame. This situation must be addressed promptly to be fair to the newly hired nurse, the preceptor, the staff, and, of course, the patients.

While it's important to understand the emotional elements involved for new graduate nurses, this does not change the fact that the level of nursing practice being displayed is unsafe and unacceptable. It is misleading to allow the new graduate to carry on believing that "things will just work out."

Key steps to take when new graduates are not progressing with critical thinking development include:

- Identifying early on those new graduates who are not meeting expectations

- Defining which expectations they are not meeting and providing examples

- Offering and providing remediation with new expectations and a written timeline for meeting the expectations

- If remediation does not change nursing practice, the manager should meet with human resources to determine the next appropriate step

For new graduates who continue to fail to progress, consider options such as these:

- Transferring the nurse, depending on his or her weaknesses, to a department outside of the pediatric unit that has

    - less-complex patients
    - fewer multitasking skills needed
    - fewer unplanned scenarios
    - lower patient-assignment loads

- Extending the probationary period

- Collaborating with faculty from his or her school of nursing for mediation direction

In all of this, do not disregard your obligations to patients and the State Board of Nursing as they relate to patient safety.

Competent to expert: Experienced nurses

Many of the principles that relate to new graduate nurses also apply to those with more experience. One of the challenges with experienced nurses is that many in the peer group have higher expectations and often believe these expectations are being met, even if they have no evidence to show this. For example, they see the experienced nurse demonstrate a particular skill or task well, and then assume all the nurse's skills are at that level. This type of assumption can be dangerous, and can mean experienced nurses receive less support and training for them to develop their critical thinking skills.

Once again, it is important to define realistic expectations for all newly hired nursing staff and establish timelines for when they should accomplish these expectations.

When experienced nurses join your unit, remind the team of the following concepts:

- Just because someone successfully completes a PALS course does not mean he or she can function in a cardiopulmonary-arrest situation

- If team members do not share concerns related to new nurse performance with the preceptor, educator, or manager, then issues cannot be addressed

- Doing a procedure faster does not imply you understand why you are doing it

- People can "talk" a great story; the test is whether they can perform at that level

- If staff nurses don't get involved in the process of orienting newly hired nurses, we cannot truly assess their abilities to think critically and act critically

In addition to experienced nurses who have just joined the unit, you should also assess and support the critical thinking development of nurses who have long been there.

Use assessment tools such as Figures 4.1, 4.2, and 5.2 to validate the ability of experienced nurses to apply critical thinking in their practice settings. For those who are unable to demonstrate their ability, initiate a remediation process in conjunction with the nurse manager.

Handling experienced nurses who need remediation

When you are confronted with seasoned nurses who are unable to meet your expectations, consider the following:

- If a new hire, do they need a different preceptor?
- If a new hire, are they still in their probationary period?
- Is there one area in which they are unable to attain a skill, or is it an overall care issue?
- If they have been staff members for a while, how has this been handled in the past?

Novice to expert: Setting realistic expectations for critical thinking

Your facility needs to use consistency when addressing this sensitive issue. If nurses are long past the orientation period and are not meeting critical-thinking expectations, find out how this has been handled with other nurses in the past. You may want to set a new precedent for how it will be handled in the future.

Because the ability to think critically is one that is ongoing and constantly being developed, it requires ongoing reevaluation. For example, just because the nurse you hired four years ago demonstrated good strategies in nursing care when he or she was hired, does not mean he or she still practices within those same principles. Consider these elements that occur in your patient care areas:

- New procedures
- New evidence and research that demonstrates a different approach to particular diagnoses
- The multitude of new medications added to the formulary each year
- New standards of practice from regulatory agencies and authorities

With this list in mind, and considering that healthcare is in constant flux, it makes sense to design a process to continually reassess nurses' ability to think critically. You can directly involve staff in this process by

- incorporating critical-thinking language and expectations in written documents such as

  - policies and procedures
  - employee handbook
  - clinical pathways/guidelines
  - job descriptions
  - performance reviews

- having staff review these written expectations annually and offer suggestions for change

- having staff complete self-assessment sheets (see Figures 4.1, 4.2, and 5.2)

- requiring staff to present examples of how they have displayed critical thinking in their patient care at their performance reviews

Measuring critical thinking in daily practice

How do you know whether nurses are thinking critically in their practice? Regardless of their level of experience, once they have completed orientation and have been "checked off" you are implying they no longer need daily precepting. You are making a statement that they have demonstrated the ability to meet their job description. If you do not feel they can perform their job description/requirements independently, then the orientation process needs to be extended.

Demonstrating they can think critically is more than being checked off on being able to perform a task or procedure. Use and adapt the sample tools throughout the book—such as Figure 4.4, which assesses their ability to think through what patients are telling them—to evaluate their level of performance. Using standard criteria for the evaluation will help you validate whether critical thinking is part of their nursing practice, for both experienced and inexperienced nurses.

Examples of demonstrating critical thinking

Pediatric nurses demonstrate critical thinking by

- identifying early signs and symptoms of dehydration in an infant with vomiting and diarrhea
- asking every parent safety questions at each visit to identify risk factors in the home environment
- evaluating attainment of developmental milestones
- asking the provider if he or she noticed the bruises on the child's extremities
- obtaining information about the family system and cultural beliefs during the assessment process
- recognizing the behavioral signs of anorexia in an adolescent female admitted for weight loss

---

Applying critical thinking to nursing documentation

LEARNING OBJECTIVE

After reading this section, the participant should be able to

- evaluate strategies to apply critical thinking to nursing documentation

Turning critical thinking into critical writing

Critical writing is as important as critical thinking. Good documentation is a vital part of patient care and nurses need to be able to validate in the written medical record what they did or what they chose not to do. We think of the medical record as a storybook that tells what happened to the patient from the point of entry into the healthcare system to the point of exit from the system. With all of today's risk management and legal concerns that challenge healthcare delivery systems as well as the caregivers, it is vital to demonstrate steps and actions taken to support the patient.

Identifying a patient problem, potential consequences, and necessary actions are vital elements of critical thinking for nurses. However, without appropriate and timely documentation, there is no written record of what has occurred.

Transforming critical thinking into the written format provides

- a legal record to support a nurse's

  - identification of a problem
  - actions taken in response to the problem
  - patient outcomes related to any intervention
  - collaboration with other members of the healthcare team
  - compliance with nursing standards of practice

- a timetable of the events to reference as a tool in determining ongoing care and needs of the patient

- validation of the nursing process that incorporated critical thinking

Figure	*Eight common charting errors*
7.1	

Accurate and complete nursing documentation is essential for demonstrating compliance with standards, delivery of state-of-the-art nursing care, and the ability to communicate effectively with everyone involved in patient care. Therefore, it is important to recognize common charting mistakes and ways to educate your staff about them.

Charting mistakes can lead to allegations of negligence. The following list describes the eight most common charting mistakes, along with how and why you should avoid them.

1. Failure to document pertinent health or drug information

Nurses conducting admission assessments are responsible for acquiring all pertinent health data that will influence the plan of care. As silly as this mistake may seem, nursing admission assessments and transfer notes are often left incomplete.

Good history-taking skills are especially important during the initial admission assessment, as the assessment is important to the safety and well-being of the patient. Any health information that is not gathered when taking the history or not documented in the appropriate location on the clinical record can lead to adverse consequences.

To avoid this kind of mistake, ensure that your staff members know how to take thorough histories and focus particularly on patients who cannot communicate effectively, are poor historians, or have dementia. Remind staff members to document conversations with significant others, the transferring agency, or any other source of information. Provide them with continuing education regarding communication skills needed to ascertain a complete and thorough patient history.

Also ensure that any important health or medication information is documented and communicated to others effectively. Neglecting to communicate an important piece of patient information can leave a nurse open to allegations of negligence. To avoid this, record the information in all of the locations designated by your policies. Also, encourage the use of bright labels and other accepted means of communicating the information.

©2007 HCPro, Inc.

Figure 7.1	Eight common charting errors (cont.)

2. Failure to record nursing actions

There needs to be a way to communicate every nursing action, and nurses must get into the habit of documenting them as close as possible to the time they occur. Unfortunately, charting is often left to the end of many nurses' busy days. This is not a good habit, but often difficult to break. Here are some guidelines to follow:

- Record all observations, assessments, and actions on the flow sheet or designated form.

- You must chart as close to the time as possible, even if it is a one- or two-line entry.

- Reduce redundancy and only chart the fact once. You do not need to repeat the same data in more than one place. Just be sure it can be found in the clinical record. If there is redundancy in your documentation system, revise it.

3. Failure to record medications given

This may seem obvious, but how many times have you reviewed a medication administration record (MAR) and found that the previous shift's nurse said in his or her report that the patient had been medicated even though you could not find it documented in the medical record?

Avoid nursing negligence by recording all medications given and the rationale for those not given, even if you may perceive them as insignificant. Always investigate when you suspect that a medication may have been administered but not recorded.

4. Recording on the wrong chart

Sometimes, a simple mistake of misfiling can lead a nurse to chart on the wrong patient. Staff are especially vulnerable to this error when patients with similar names are on the same unit, so you need a system of identification that is clear and as foolproof as possible.

Figure	
7.1	*Eight common charting errors (cont.)*

Errors in this category include

- transcribing medication orders onto the wrong patient's chart.

- writing progress notes without confirming the accuracy of the chart you chose. To prevent this error, look at the external name on the chart and always look at the name stamped at the top of the document.

Whenever possible, do not assign the same nurse to patients with the same name. And always ensure compliance with the National Patient Safety Goal that refers to proper patient identification prior to procedures and medication administration.

5. Failure to document a discontinued medication

Nurses are responsible for ensuring safe patient care at all levels. When a medication has been ordered to be discontinued, the change must be appropriately noted according to policy and communicated to the next shift's nurse. Nurses also need to comply with the organization's policies concerning cross-checking the physician orders with the MAR. Doing so can prevent serious complications.

6. Failure to document drug reactions/changes in patient's condition

The literature on "failure to rescue" points to this potential error. Nurses are responsible for the assessment of a patient's reaction to medication and for the identification of any change in a patient's condition. They must have the skill and knowledge to anticipate the clinical needs of a patient. They must also possess critical thinking skills to intervene appropriately in any adverse reaction or worsening of the patient's condition. But performing this assessment, identification, and intervention is not enough. Nurses must also document that they have done so.

Figure	
7.1	*Eight common charting errors (cont.)*

7. Improper transcription of orders or transcription of improper orders

The registered nurse can be held liable for transcribing improper doses that led to a patient's injury. The nurse can also be held liable for transcribing and carrying out an order they know to be inaccurate or suspect to be incorrect.

If the nurses discuss both the order and their concerns with physicians, they must document these conversations. In addition, if nurses still maintain that administration of the medication or proceeding with a procedure is not in the best interest of the patient, they must activate the chain of command and document that as well.

In contemporary nursing practice, all nurses must know medications or research a new medication prior to administration. If a nurse is not familiar with a procedure and does not seek supervision or assistance with it, questions of clinical competence and ensuring patient safety will come into play if there is any question of malpractice. The public expects that we will continue to keep our professional skills and knowledge up to date. Falling short of this will put a nurse in a difficult position from which to defend her- or himself.

8. Writing illegible or incomplete records

Illegible handwriting is no longer tolerated by regulatory and accreditation surveyors. With the goal of improving patient safety, the days of laughing at someone's handwriting are over. All providers who document in the clinical record must ensure that what they have written is readable. Should the clinical record be reviewed, it is essential that the author of the record be able to clearly read it. Some hospitals have instituted illegible handwriting policies to improve compliance with legible-documentation standards and to improve patient safety.

Source: DuClos-Miller, P. 2004. Managing Documentation Risk: A Guide for Nurse Managers. *Marblehead, MA: HCPro, Inc.*

Examples of critical writing skills

The following are examples of the application of critical writing skills.

Patient case 1

One night in early January, you are floated to the pediatric unit at a small community hospital that also cares for overflow adult patients from the surgical unit. You worked on this unit two years ago before transferring to the nursery. Tonight, the charge nurse called in sick, and the supervisor asked you to be in charge. The unit has 20 beds, and often is less than half full. During the winter months, however, the unit is filled with pediatric patients. On this particular night shift there are 18 pediatric patients with one additional admission expected from the emergency department. The staff for the shift consists of one new graduate RN, two LPNs, and one nursing assistant.

1915	Entered room 403 to investigate a parent complaint reported by the nursing supervisor during change of shift report. Entered the room to find the mother asleep in the chair and the 9-month-old patient lying in the bed whimpering and lethargic. As the crib rails are lowered, the mother awakens and says, "Please do something for my baby. He is so sick, and the doctor hasn't been in to see him since early this morning. I am so worried about him, and nobody seems to be doing anything to help him."
1916	After completing a head to toe assessment, findings include a weak cry, dry mucous membranes, clammy skin, and a diffuse petechial rash. HR 140, respirations 40, and temperature 103 degrees F.
1917	Paged Resident on call stat to patient's room. Nursing supervisor notified. Patient's mother at patient's side crying. Notified LPN to watch other patients, and stayed with child and mom until physician arrived.
1922	Physician arrived to examine patient. Explained diagnostic procedures to patient's mother and asked RN to accompany him to treatment room to assist with work-up.
1935	Blood cultures and lumbar puncture completed. Intravenous fluids and antibiotic therapy initiated. Patient transferred to ICU for close observation.

The documentation shows that the pediatric nurse exhibited autonomy and responsibility. He or she exhibited independent thinking and actions in assessing the patient, realizing the seriousness of the situation, and notifying the Resident on call to urgently see the patient.

The nurse was also proactive by staying with the patient and his mother until the physician arrived and notifying the LPN to monitor the other patients.

Patient case 2

The pediatric nurse admits a two-year-old male with history of a fall from his crib and a suspected skull fracture.

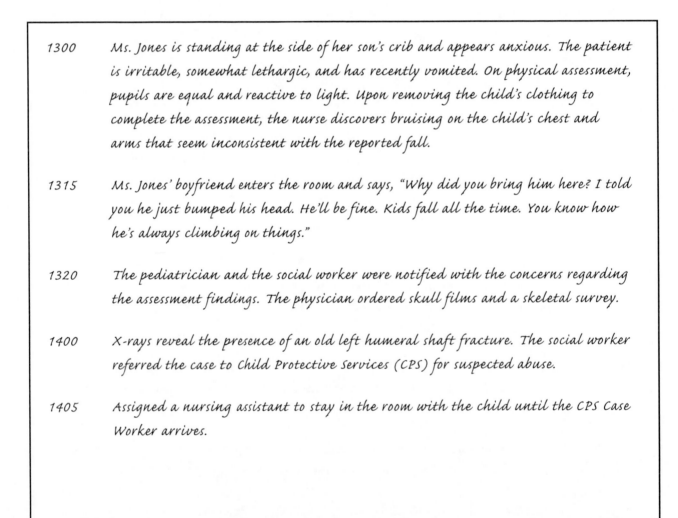

1300	Ms. Jones is standing at the side of her son's crib and appears anxious. The patient is irritable, somewhat lethargic, and has recently vomited. On physical assessment, pupils are equal and reactive to light. Upon removing the child's clothing to complete the assessment, the nurse discovers bruising on the child's chest and arms that seem inconsistent with the reported fall.
1315	Ms. Jones' boyfriend enters the room and says, "Why did you bring him here? I told you he just bumped his head. He'll be fine. Kids fall all the time. You know how he's always climbing on things."
1320	The pediatrician and the social worker were notified with the concerns regarding the assessment findings. The physician ordered skull films and a skeletal survey.
1400	X-rays reveal the presence of an old left humeral shaft fracture. The social worker referred the case to Child Protective Services (CPS) for suspected abuse.
1405	Assigned a nursing assistant to stay in the room with the child until the CPS Case Worker arrives.

 ©2007 HCPro, Inc.   **Critical Thinking in the Pediatric Unit**

The pediatric nurse used critical thinking skills by completing a physical assessment and questioning findings that seemed inconsistent with the history of the child's fall. The nurse was proactive in communicating her findings and concerns to the physician and the social worker. The critical thinking skills used by the nurse are both logical and intuitive. The nurse used sound judgment in identifying and communicating her concerns and working with the multidisciplinary team to expedite appropriate evaluation and referrals.

Patient case 3

The nurse is caring for a four-year-old girl with a history of back pain, high fever, and frequent, painful urination.

0920	On entering Room 645, the patient is found to be irritable and crying intermittently for her mother, who is at work and will not be able to visit until late afternoon. Unable to comfort child by reading a story or attempting to engage her in play activities.
0921	Upon completing a brief assessment, observed that her panties, pajamas, and bed pad were soaked with blood-tinged urine. After weighing the pad and clothing and recording the output, reviewed the orders and medication record to determine what medications could be given to alleviate her pain. She had acetaminophen ordered every 4 hours by mouth for pain and/or fever greater than 101 degrees F. The night nurse had given her the last dose at 0715 for an elevated temperature of 102 degrees. When assessing her pain using the Faces Pain Scale, her pain score was 3.
0923	Pediatrician was contacted to inform her of the hematuria and to request additional pain medication for the patient.
0935	Dr. Brown at bedside to examine patient. New orders written for renal ultrasound, a Urology consult, and acetaminophen with codeine elixir (120 mg acetaminophen and 12 mg codeine per 5 ml). 10 ml now and every 4 hours for pain.
0940	The first dose of acetaminophen with codeine elixir obtained from pharmacy and administered.

 ©2007 HCPro, Inc.

> 1015   Before calling the child's mother at work to provide an update, went to check on patient and found her sleeping comfortably. Reported the child's status, reviewed new physician orders, and let the mom know that the physician would provide a comprehensive update for her this afternoon when she arrived to see her daughter after work.

The pediatric nurse exhibits critical thinking skills by collecting the data needed to make an evidence-based assessment. The nurse is proactive and demonstrates an understanding of the use of age-appropriate non-pharmacologic pain management to initially attempt managing the child's pain. The nurse is analytical in investigating the child's pharmacologic pain management and recognizing that the medication ordered did not effectively manage the child's pain. The nurse displays sensitivity to the mother's needs by contacting her to provide an update. The nurse is careful and prudent to evaluate the effectiveness of her intervention in managing the child's pain and report the new finding of hematuria to the physician.

Patient case 4

The pediatric nurse is caring for a 10-year-old patient with asthma.

> 1036   Entered patient's room to complete assessment and hang a new bag of IV fluids. Patient's parents were present, and asked if there was an area where they could go outside to smoke. They were directed to the smoking area and informed that RN will look in on their son while they were out.
>
> 1045   Upon hanging the new bag of IV fluids and completing the assessment, the patient is found to have nasal flaring, coarse breath sounds, and bilateral wheezing.
>
> Went back to talk with parents and questioned them regarding their smoking habits and whether they smoked in the home. They both answered that they smoked in the house. This was their child's third hospital admission for asthma in the past year. Asked if anyone had given them information about the effects of second hand smoke, and they said their pediatrician had told them not to smoke around their son.

    ©2007 HCPro, Inc.   **Critical Thinking in the Pediatric Unit**

> 1115   *Went to the patient education file, obtained some educational materials for the parents regarding "smoking and asthma," and reviewed the materials with the parents. Also contacted the Respiratory Therapist to join RN in spending some time with the family reviewing home management of asthma and available community resources.*

The nurse demonstrates critical thinking by recognizing the effect of the parents' smoking habits on their child's asthma and repeated hospital admissions. Without passing judgment on the parents, the nurse proactively involves another multidisciplinary team member in educating the parents about the effects of smoking on asthma and providing information regarding community resources to assist in managing their child's asthma. The nurse's educational interventions are designed to help this family improve asthma management at home and reduce the need for hospital admissions.

Relating critical thinking to its higher purpose

In nursing, we tend to work toward achieving goals as the end of a process, when many times meeting the goal is just the beginning. In this book, Polly Gerber Zimmermann reminds us that *learning to think critically is a journey, not a destination.* The foundation of critical thinking skills you build for nurses will be directly reflected in your ability to continue on this path. The ability to meet the needs of our patients is a moving walkway that seems to go on forever. Each specialty of healthcare delivery is faced with having to provide care to more patients at a faster pace with fewer resources.

Whether you work in acute care, rehab, home health, or medical-office settings, or in any other environment, nurses are the people patients and families turn to. They turn to us for clarification, guidance, hope, and the truth.

While driving home from the hospital, I was listening to a postal worker in New Orleans being interviewed on public radio. The postal worker was delivering mail to a district recently reopened after Hurricane Katrina. The interview went along these lines:

Q: What kind of challenges are you facing with this delivery area?
A: Well, there are lots of challenges, such as the debris and trash.

Q: Is it difficult to tell whether or not it is the right house you are delivering to?
*A: If the number is no longer there or the mailbox is gone we are supposed to use **deductive reasoning** to determine if it is the right house. For example, I might look to see if it is a consecutive number.*

Critical Thinking in the Pediatric Unit

©2007 HCPro, Inc.

This interview reminds us that we use critical thinking in our daily lives without realizing it. For example we think critically

- at the grocery store to determine if the sale price is really a sale or just a cheaper price on a smaller container

- when our child tells us, "I did study for that exam," yet you never saw a book in his or her room

- at the dentist office when we decide whether to pay to fix the tooth or have it pulled

We cannot continue to improve the quality of care we deliver without engaging our reasoning. The ability to reason and consider actions or inactions is a feature of critical thinking that provides a safe patient-care environment. Recognizing the best interest of the patient is paramount in quality-improvement processes. As you consider all of the efforts in which your organization is engaged regarding meeting regulatory standards remember this:

Staff members cannot meet the needs of patients if they cannot recognize those needs.

Resources and tools

This chapter contains additional tools and resources to assist you in assessing and developing pediatric nurses' critical thinking capabilities at the point of hire, during orientation, and through ongoing development and review. This chapter contains

- a list of further reading and resources

- additional sample questions

- Figure 9.1, which is a handout that can be given to attendees of a critical thinking class who want further information and study materials

- Figure 9.2, which contains unfolding teaching scenarios that can be used for discussing critical thinking

- Figure 9.3, which contains examples of teachable moments

- Figure 9.4, which contains additional pediatric case studies

- Figure 9.5, which is a sample critical thinking–skills class agenda that can be customized for any facility

- Figures 9.6–9.12, which are worksheets that can be used or adapted for critical thinking classes, during orientation, or for ongoing critical thinking development.

Resources and further reading

Online publications

National Heart, Lung, and Blood Institute. 2006. "Diseases and Conditions Index: Asthma." Accessed from *www.nhlbi.nih.gov/health/dci/Diseases/Asthma/Asthma_WhatIs.html*.

University of Michigan Health System. "Pain Management Staff Development Education—Part 5: Pediatric Pain Management." Accessed from *www.med.umich.edu/pain/pediatric.htm*.

The Pediatric Orthopaedic Society of North America. 2006. "Fractures of the humeral shaft." *In Core Curriculum*. Accessed from *www.posna.org/index?service=page/coreCurriculum*.

American Academy of Allergy, Asthma & Immunology. 2002. "Resources: Pediatric Asthma: Promoting Best Practices." Accessed from *www.aaaai.org/members/resources/initiatives/pediatricasthmaguidelines/default.stm*.

Publications

Buck, M.L. 2004. "Therapeutic uses of codeine in pediatric patients." *Pediatric Pharmacology* 12 (6): 1. Children's Medical Center of the University of Virginia.

Hockenberry, M., ed. 2004. *Clinical Manual of Pediatric Nursing*. 6th ed. St. Louis, MO: Mosby.

Hockenberry, M., ed. 2005. *Essentials of Pediatric Nursing*. 7th ed. St. Louis, MO: Mosby.

Manworren, R. and Hynan, L. 2003. "Clinical validation of FLACC: Preverbal patient pain scale." *Pediatric Nursing* 29 (2): 140-146.

Wong, D. and Baker, C. 1988. "Pain in children: Comparison of assessment scales." *Pediatric Nursing*. 14 (1): 9017.

General nursing and critical thinking

Alfaro-Lefevre, R. 2004. Critical Thinking and Clinical Judgment: A Practical Approach. St Louis, MO: Saunders.

Doan-Johnson, S. and A. Woods, eds. 2005. *Nursing Made Incredibly Easy*. Philadelphia: Lippincott Williams & Wilkins.

DuClos-Miller, P. 2004. *Managing Documentation Risk: A Guide for Nurse Managers*. Marblehead, MA: HCPro, Inc.

Goodman, B. 2006. "How to ask an intelligent question." *Nursing Standard* 20 (24): 81.

Haggerty, L. A. and R. L. Nuttall. 2000. "Experienced obstetric nurses' decision-making in fetal risk situations." *Journal of Obstetric, Gynecologic, & Neonatal Nursing* 29 (5): 480-490.

Hsu, L. and S. Hsieh. 2005. "Concept maps as an assessment tool in a nursing course." *Journal of Professional Nursing* 21 (3):141-149.

Lauri, S., S. Salantera, K. Chalmers, S. Ekmann, S. Hesook, S. Kappeli and M. MacLeod. 2001. "An exploratory study of clinical decision-making in five countries." *Journal of Nursing Scholarship* 33 (1): 83-90.

Lipe, S. K. and S. Beasley. 2004. *Critical Thinking in Nursing: A Cognitive Skills Workbook*. Philadelphia: Lippincott Williams & Wilkins.

Myrick, F. and O. Yonge. 2002. "Preceptor questioning and student thinking." *Journal of Professional Nursing* 18 (3):176-181.

Profetto-McGrath, J. 2005. "Critical thinking and evidence-based practice." *Journal of Professional Nursing* 21 (6):364-371.

Rubenfeld, M. G. and B. K. Scheffer. 2006. *Critical Thinking Tactics for Nurses*. Sudbury, MA: Jones and Bartlett.

Scheffer, B. K. 2006. "Critical thinking: A tool in search of a job." *Journal of Nursing Education* 45 (6):195-196.

Springhouse. 2004. *Nurses Legal Handbook*. Philadelphia: Lippincott Williams & Wilkins.

Springhouse. 2006. *Professional Guide to Signs & Symptoms*, 5th ed. Philadelphia: Lippincott Williams & Wilkins.

Tanner, C. A. 2006. "Thinking like a nurse: A research-based model of clinical judgment in nursing." *Journal of Nursing Education* 45 (6): 204-211.

Thompson, C. 2001. "Clinical decision making in nursing: Theoretical perspectives and their relevance to practice—a response to Jean Harbison." *Journal of Advanced Nursing* 35 (1), 134-137.

Wright, D. 1998. *The Ultimate Guide to Competency Assessment in Healthcare*. Eau Claire, WI: PESI Healthcare.

Yocum, Fay. 1999. *Documentation Skills for Quality Patient Care*. Dayton, OH: Awareness Productions.

Zunkel, G. M., E. L. Cesarotti, D. Rosdahl and J. M. McGrath. 2004. "Enhancing diagnostic reasoning skills in nurse practitioner students: A teaching tool." *Nurse Educator* 29 (4): 161-165.

Pediatric nurse as researcher

Banning, M. 2006. "Nursing research: Perspectives on critical thinking." *British Journal of Nursing* 15 (8): 458-461.

Brink, P. J. and M. J. Wood. 1994. *Basic Steps in Planning Nursing Research: From Question to Proposal*. 4th ed. Boston: Jones and Bartlett Publishers.

Cultural diversity

Giger, J. N. 1995. *Transcultural Nursing: Assessment and Intervention*. St Louis, MO: Mosby.

Spector, R. E. 1991. *Cultural Diversity in Health and Illness*. 3rd ed. East Norwalk, CT: Appleton-Century Crofts.

Web sites

Enchanted Learning: *www.enchantedlearning.com*
- Anatomy diagrams/glossaries and more

North Central Regional Educational Laboratory (NCREL®): *www.ncrel.org*
- Resources defining critical thinking

The Advisory Board Company: *www.advisory.com*
- Multiple resources: Search under new graduate nurse

National Council of State Boards of Nursing: *www.ncsbn.org*
- Access to all state Boards of Nursing rules and regulations

Perinatal Continuing Education Program: *www.pcep.org*
- Site for the Perinatal Continuing Education Program for physicians, nurses, and all others who care for pregnant women or newborn babies

The Institute for Family-Centered Care: *www.familycenteredcare.org*
- Promotes collaboration between care provider and family, offering educational material and other professional resources for family-centered care at home and in the hospital

Society of Pediatric Nurses: *www.PedsNurses.org*
- Professional association for nurses caring for children

Healthy People 2010: *www.HealthyPeople.gov*
- Federally funded series of national health objectives that aims to identify preventable threats to health and set goals to reduce them; look for professional resources including sections on the Best Practice Initiative, Implementations, and Leading Health Indicators

American Nurses Association: *www.NursingWorld.org*
- Information on many issues facing the professional nurse today

National Association of Pediatric Nurse Practitioners: *www.napnap.org*
- Resource for pediatric nurse practitioners and nurses to promote children's health through advocacy, education, and research

American Academy of Nurse Practitioners: *www.AANP.org*
- Resource for nurse practitioners to promote excellence in practice, education, and research

Foundation for Critical Thinking: *www.criticalthinking.org*
- Non-profit organization that works to promote educational reform and promote critical thinking; non-healthcare specific

Additional sample questions

Source: June Marshall, RN, MS, CNAA,BC

These questions may be used either for discussion or for a test. Remove answers before providing them to learners. (File can be found under "Additional sample questions" on the accompanying CD-ROM.)

Question: The patient is post-op day two following a pyloromyotomy, is bottle feeding, and is scheduled to be discharged this morning. The nurse examines the patient and finds the patient's abdomen distended and firm, and the patient has vomited twice this shift. The patient's skin is hot and the baby is irritable. The patient has had no bowel movement since the procedure. Patient's mom complains that the baby has been straining and crying out after feedings like he is trying to have a bowel movement. What is the first action the nurse should take?

    a. Take the patient's vital signs

    b. Medicate the patient for pain

    c. Start discharge instructions

    d. Notify the physician immediately

Answer: D

The nurse should notify the physician immediately. The patient's mom's complaints and the child's physical assessment are significant for possible postoperative complications and need immediate follow-up by the physician.

Through using critical thinking, the nurse knows that the patient's abdominal distension and vomiting may be signs of constipation or an intestinal obstruction. The child's warm skin temperature may indicate a postoperative infection. The child cannot be discharged until these problems are evaluated and resolved.

Question: When performing a physical exam of a newborn, which of the following should the nurse report to the provider immediately?

   a. Patent anterior fontanel
   b. Head circumference 4cm less than chest circumference
   c. Positive Babinski sign
   d. Cyanosis of the hands and feet

Answer: B

Circumference of the head should be 2cm greater than the circumference of the newborn's chest at birth and will remain in this proportion for the next few months.

Question: The patient has an epidural catheter in place and received her first dose of medication for postoperative pain 1 hour ago. The nurse takes the patient's blood pressure and pulse and observes a change in blood pressure from 110/60 to 128/80 and a change in pulse from 86 to 94. The nurse's first action should be to

   a. notify the physician
   b. check the epidural catheter and dressing to ensure that the catheter has not become dislodged and is not leaking
   c. review the orders and medication record to assess that the patient received the appropriate dose of medication
   d. question the parents about the child's pain tolerance

Answer: B

The nurse should use critical thinking and apply his or her knowledge of physiology to the change in the patient's condition. This means the nurse will think about what is causing the change in vital signs and what the meaning of such a change could be.

The nurse's first action should be to check the epidural catheter to ensure correct placement and functioning. The nurse should then check the orders to ensure the medication dose is appropriate for the child's age and weight.

If everything is in order, the nurse should contact the physician, report the change in vital signs, and ask to adjust the dose of medication, since it is not relieving the patient's pain. Until the physician arrives to change the dose, the nurse should try to use non-pharmacologic methods of pain relief to assist the child in managing the pain until additional medication can be given.

Question: The patient is a 12-year-old child with spina bifida at the lumbar level that was admitted for 2nd degree scald burns to both feet. The burns are healing nicely, and the parents have successfully performed all of the wound care several times. The child is ready for discharge and can return to school as well. What is the most important action to prevent future injuries in this child?

    a. Have the parents supervise all the patient's care
    b. Teach the child how to protect his skin from temperatures that are too hot/cold
    c. Wear protective clothing at school when playing wheelchair sports
    d. Keep the skin moist with daily application of lotion

Answer: B

Critical thinking involves inquisitiveness, so the nurse should question what caused this injury, and what steps can be taken to prevent future injuries. The nurse knows that children with spina bifida at the lumbar level have little or absent sensation below the level of the lesion. The nurse also knows that injuries from excessive heat and cold can do more damage to someone without sensation, since they do not react in the same way as those with normal sensation.

The nurse also knows that helping a 12-year-old be independent in self-care is important for healthy growth and development. Therefore, the nurse will focus on teaching the important aspects of self-care and injury prevention to this patient, while also reinforcing aspects of this teaching with the patient's parents.

Question: The unit has not received an advance call from the emergency department or admissions that a patient is on the way up, but the doors to the unit have just flown open. The emergency medical technicians (EMT) rush in a litter upon which is a patient in respiratory distress who had just been discharged yesterday. What is the nurse's first course of action and why?

a. Thank the EMTs for the surprise as it had been a slow day up until then
b. Take the patient's vital signs and begin the admission assessment
c. Notify the physician of the patient's arrival
d. Ask the patient's mom when she last ate

Answer: B

Inexperienced nurses may be hesitant to take immediate action to examine the patient in acute distress. However, it is of primary importance to know the patient's current status before contacting the physician.

Critical thinkers are forward moving, show independent thinking, and take responsibility for their actions. They should not be timid about taking immediate action.

<table>
<tr><td>Figure

9.1</td><td>Critical thinking skills course—
Additional resources handout</td></tr>
</table>

■ **Dorothy Del Bueno's article about critical thinking displayed by nurses:**

Del Bueno, D. 2001. "Buyer beware: The cost of competence." *Nursing Economics* 19 (6): 259–257.

■ **American Association of Critical-Care Nursing (AACN) decision tree for delegation decisions:** Available from 101 Columbia, Alisa Viejo, CA 92656-1491; 800/899-2226

■ **Give new graduates "rules" for "telling somebody" by using the criteria developed for Rapid Response Team Activation** (a concept introduced by the Institute for Healthcare Improvement [IHI] as part of the "100,000 Lives Campaign.")

- IHI recommendations: *www.ihi.org/IHI/Programs/TransformingCareattheBedside*.

- Scholle, C. C., and C. Mininni. 2006 "Best-practice interventions: How a Rapid Response Team saves lives." *Nursing2006* 36 (1): 36–40.

  – Mean arterial pressure < 70 or > 130 mmHg
  – Heart rate < 45 or > 125
  – Respiratory rate < 10 or > 30
  – Complaints of chest pain
  – Change in mental status (lasting more than 10 minutes)

According to one study, 66% of patients had signs of instability for up to eight hours prior to the event. Studies have shown that up to 70% of the calls to a Rapid Response Team were based on concerns about the patient's respiratory status, accompanied by staff concern about a patient's deteriorating condition.

Figure	*Critical thinking skills course—*
9.1	*Additional resources handout (cont.)*

■ **"Brains in our Pocket" resources for nurses**

- PDA programs

    - See Audrey Snyder's chapter "PDA Use" in P. G. Zimmermann and R. D. Herr, 2006, *Triage Nursing Secrets* (St. Louis: Mosby/Elsevier) for suggested programs and sources to obtain them.

- Print:

    - Myers, E. 2003. *RNotes: Nurse's Clinical Pocket Guide*. Philadelphia: FA Davis.

■ **Good sources of test questions**

- LaCharity, L. A, C. D. Kumagai, and B. Bartz. 2005. *Prioritization, Delegation & Assignment Practice Exercises for Medical-Surgical Nursing*. St. Louis: Mosby/Elsevier.

- Springhouse. 2006. *NCLEX-RN: 250 New-Format Questions*. Philadelphia: Lippincott Williams & Wilkins.

- Rayfield, S., and L. Manning. 2004. *NCLEX-RN 101: How to Pass!*, 5th ed. Gulf Shores, AL: ICAN.

■ **Aids for writing better test questions**

- Bosher, S. 2003. "Linguistic bias in multiple-choice nursing exams." *Nursing Education Perspectives* 24 (1): 25–34.

- Zimmermann, P. G. 2005. "Writing effective test questions." *Journal of Emergency Nursing* 32 (1): 106–109.

■ **Concept mapping**

- Carpenito-Moyet, L. J. 2005. *Understanding the Nursing Process: Concept Mapping and Care Planning for Students*. Philadelphia: Lippincott Williams & Wilkins.

<table>
<tr><td>Figure
9.1</td><td>Critical thinking skills course—
Additional resources handout (cont.)</td></tr>
</table>

- Schuster, P. M. 2000. "Concept mapping: Reducing clinical care plan paperwork and increasing learning." *Nurse Educator* 25 (2): 76–81.

■ Critical thinking books

- Rubenfeld, M. G., and B. K. Scheffer. 2006. *Critical Thinking Tactics for Nurses.* Sudbury, MA: Jones and Bartlett.

- Lipe, S. K., and S. Beasley. 2004. *Critical Thinking in Nursing: A Cognitive Skills Workbook.* Philadelphia: Lippincott Williams & Wilkins.

■ Generation X/multigeneration work force

- Duchscher, J. E. B., and L. Cowin. 2004. "Multigenerational nurses in the workplace." *Journal of Nursing Administration* 34 (11): 493–501.

- Lower, J. 2006. *A Practical Guide to Managing the Multigenerational Workforce: Skills for Nurse Managers.* Marblehead, MA: HCPro.

- Raines, C. 2002. "Managing Generation X Employees" in P. G. Zimmermann's *Nursing Management Secrets.* Philadelphia: Hanley & Belfus.

- Raines, C. 1997. *Beyond Generation X.* Menlo Park, CA: Crisp.

- Sacks, P. 1996. *Generation X Goes to College.* Chicago and LaSalle, IL: Open Court.

■ Example of a worst-case scenario

- Zimmermann, P. G. (2003) "Lessons learned: On watching for zebras." *Journal of Emergency Nursing* 29 (1): 85–86.

Source: Polly Gerber Zimmermann, RN, MS, MBA, CEN

Figure

9.2

Unfolding teaching scenarios for pediatric nurses

These scenarios can be used as discussion areas during critical thinking classes or adapted and given to nurses for further reading.

Scenario 1

Who-When-What-Think-Ask-Do

Who: 2-year-old male admitted with history of weight loss

When: Hospital day 1

What: Mother states, "He just seems tired all the time and doesn't even want to play. I'm really worried about him."

New graduate nurse thinks:

"Oh no, this could be childhood cancer."

REMEMBER

Having a little bit of knowledge can be a dangerous thing. Don't draw conclusions without enough facts.

Think: There are a number of causes of weight loss in young children. The pediatrician is obtaining all of the necessary diagnostic studies to determine the child's diagnosis, and I need to focus on assessing the child and gathering the facts. The physician admission note includes Type I Diabetes as part of the differential diagnosis.

Ask: How much urine/stool output is he having? He has been urinating large amounts of urine and having firm bowel movements every other day, according to his mother.

Is the child in pain? No, his FLACC Pain Scale score is 0.

What is the child's food/fluid intake? He has been unusually thirsty and has a normal appetite.

Does he have any other symptoms?

Is his height and weight normal for age or has he fallen off the normal growth curve?

> **Figure 9.2** — *Unfolding teaching scenarios for pediatric nurses (cont.)*

Do: **Observe/Assess:**

Skin: Turgor, temperature, rashes, wounds, bruising, etc. Skin is dry and flaky.

Neurological status: Lethargy, mental status, muscle tone. Somewhat lethargic.

Vital signs: Temperature, heart rate, and respirations for any abnormalities. WNL.

Intake and output: Oral intake and urine/stool output to evaluate hydration and nutritional status.

Developmental milestones for age.

Diagnose (once diagnosis of Type I Diabetes has been confirmed):

Knowledge deficit—home management of Type I Diabetes

Intervene:

Provide parent(s) with individualized education regarding home management of diabetes as outlined by the diabetes educator and nutritionist and establish plan for home care and follow-up on discharge.

Scenario 2

Who-When-What-Think-Ask-Do

Who: The emergency department (ED) calls to report that a 10-year-old female in respiratory distress, discharged from your unit last week, is en route to the hospital via ambulance. The ED is very busy. After a brief evaluation, the patient will be admitted directly to your unit to avoid a long wait in the ED.

When the patient arrives and a brief evaluation confirms the need for admission, you are given report by the ED nurse.

When: The patient's parents only speak Spanish. The patient was sent home from school earlier in the day. By the time her father arrived home from work to transport her to the hospital, she had severe wheezing that was unresponsive to her routine medication regimen. The mother is visibly upset with the father, and the patient is growing increasingly anxious.

 ©2007 HCPro, Inc.   **Critical Thinking in the Pediatric Unit**

Figure	*Unfolding teaching scenarios*
9.2	*for pediatric nurses (cont.)*

What: You prepare to assist the admitting physician to get her IV started, obtain her labs, administer oxygen, and perform her admission assessment. You settle her parents in the room, while you and the physician take the patient to the treatment room.

What is your first action?

REMEMBER

Think before acting. Respond to the situation without reacting to it.

Think: What do I need to do to provide this patient and her family a smooth admission and a safe, effective hospitalization?

Ask: How can I communicate with this family and help them understand the importance of effective asthma management at home without showing frustration over this patient's frequent readmissions?

Do: Because you cannot speak Spanish, you move forward quickly to admit the patient and assist the physician, while asking the unit coordinator to contact the translator on call.

Quickly move to address the patient's immediate needs.

When the IV is started, the labs are drawn, the medications are given, and the patient is breathing more comfortably, then the parent session can be initiated with the translator present to assist.

Ensure that comprehensive education and plans for home management and outpatient follow-up are priorities for this hospital stay.

INSTRUCTOR:
- Prompt students to think why these specific actions are important.
- If no response, prompt application of knowledge of asthma triggers and any cultural implications involved in adherence to home management regimen.
- Guide the students through the steps involved in prevention of acute exacerbations, asthma treatment protocols, and management of respiratory distress.
- Discuss transcultural nursing and transcultural caring.

| Figure 9.2 | Unfolding teaching scenarios for pediatric nurses (cont.) |

Scenario 3

Who-When-What-Think-Ask-Do

Who, When, What: You are a pool nurse assigned to 4-East, the pediatric medical unit. The unit has had an overwhelming number of admissions in the past 24 hours and you are assigned there for this shift.

Your assignment is as follows:

Patient 1: B.J.

6 months old

RSV

Hospital day 2

Febrile

Congested

Patient 2: S.T.

14 years old

Cystic Fibrosis

Hospital day 1

Respiratory distress

Vomiting

Febrile

Frequent respiratory treatments

Patient 3: T.M.

2 years old

Urinary tract infection

Hospital day 2

Febrile

Frequent voiding

Having severe pain

Parents unable to stay with patient

Figure

9.2

Unfolding teaching scenarios for pediatric nurses (cont.)

Patient 4: J.K.

12 years old

Type 2 Diabetes

Hospital Day 1

Ketoacidosis

Father is an attorney

Parents are very demanding and question every action

Patient 5: N.R.

10 months old

Failure to thrive

Hospital day 10

IV TPN via central venous catheter

Parents divorced, and father does not have custody

Father has history of violence and tries to see patient

After receiving report you feel overwhelmed and think this assignment may be more than you can handle since you are called to this unit less frequently than the surgical pediatric unit. You also realize that the unit nurses are carrying heavy patient loads due to the increased census and short staff situation.

What do you do?

INSTRUCTOR:

- Ask students for possible actions this nurse can take
- Discuss the ethics of this situation with the students
- Relate this situation to "knowing what you don't know"

REMEMBER

Fear of the unknown can rob you of your power.

| Figure 9.2 | Unfolding teaching scenarios for pediatric nurses (cont.) |

Think: What does my assignment actually entail? Break it down and put it in perspective.

1. Hospital day 2, RSV, febrile and congested
2. Hospital day 1, CF, respiratory distress, vomiting, febrile, frequent respiratory treatments
3. Hospital day 2, UTI, febrile, frequent voiding, pain, parents absent
4. Hospital day 1, Type 2 Diabetes, ketoacidosis, demanding parents
5. Hospital day 10, failure to thrive, TPN, security issues

Ask: Now that the assignment is put into perspective, does it still look unmanageable? Reassess.

- Do I feel comfortable with this assignment?
- If I still don't feel comfortable with the assignment do I have any options? What exactly are those options?
- Am I willing to exercise those options with the potential for appearing to be less of a "team player" to my peers?
- Is there anything unethical or illegal about any of my options?
- Will I accept the assignment even if I feel unsure about my ability to provide safe care for all my patients?

Do: Take action on your decision. What are the possible actions you could take?

- Notify supervisor to discuss concerns
- Accept assignment
- Refuse assignment
- Accept assignment under duress
- Ask for a different assignment
- Share assignment with a regular staff member on that unit

Source: June Marshall, RN, MS, CNAA,BC

Figure 9.3	*Pediatric unit teachable moments*

Case 1

Who-When-What-Think-Ask-Do

Who, what, when: You are assigned to the day shift and you are caring for a 6-month-old neurologically impaired infant with failure to thrive. The infant has gained weight receiving NG feedings and is being discharged to home with foster parents. You have been given report that discharge teaching was provided to the foster parents during the night shift. You have read the night shift nurse's notes that state she gave discharge instructions to the parents.

Think: What is your next course of action?

Ask: Am I sure and am I able to document that I discharged this foster family to home with full discharge instructions and that they know how to care for this infant?

REMEMBER
When in doubt about a course of action to be taken, think about what questions would be asked of you, and how you would answer them, if they were being asked by an attorney or an ethicist.

Do: Ask questions that reveal the caregiver's level of understanding of the discharge teaching:

- Are the caregivers able to feed the infant via the NG tube and assess tolerance of the enteral feeding regimen?
- Do the caregivers have a written instruction sheet including the phone number of a contact person they can call to report problems or to ask further questions?
- Do the caregivers know WHEN and for WHAT situations to call the contact person?
- If presented with a hypothetical scenario, do the caregivers respond with the appropriate action to be taken for the situation?

Figure	
9.3	*Pediatric unit teachable moments (cont.)*

Document your assurance that you are discharging this family to home and that they are capable of caring for this infant.

REMEMBER

Even though discharge instructions were given during the night shift, **you** are the nurse who is releasing this patient and foster family from the care of the hospital.

Case 2

Who-When-What-Think-Ask-Do

Who, what, when: The nurse is assigned to the gastroenterology clinic attached to the pediatric acute care hospital. A 14-year-old patient diagnosed with ulcerative colitis arrives for her regular follow-up visit after being discharged from the hospital two weeks ago. She complains of increased bloody diarrhea and rectal and abdominal pain.

Think: The nurse **recognizes** that the patient's complaints of rectal pain may be associated with an exacerbation of her ulcerative colitis and rectal ulcers.

Ask: How should I **prioritize** my care?

Do: The nurse **positions** the patient in the left lateral recumbent position before assessing the skin around her anal opening. The nurse also observes that the patient's abdomen is distended.

The nurse **anticipates** the provider's orders and contacts personnel in the outpatient laboratory and in radiology to let them know they need to stay late to accommodate this patient's diagnostic evaluation.

Figure 9.3	*Pediatric unit teachable moments (cont.)*

The nurse **instructs** the patient and family about possible next steps, while they wait for the gastroenterologist.

The patient is seen by the provider and orders are written for the patient to be admitted for a suspected intestinal perforation.

In calling report to the GI unit and documenting the clinic visit, the nurse includes the following:

"14-year-old female patient of Dr. Jones with the diagnosis of ulcerative colitis to R/O intestinal perforation to be admitted to 5-North.

Chief complaint rectal and abdominal pain, bloody diarrhea, and perianal ulcers increasing in severity over the last 48 hours, poor appetite, and nausea without vomiting.

+Abdominal distention and diffuse tenderness
+Perianal ulcers at 6:00 and 10:00
+Anal fissures
+Hemocult stool

Labs drawn for Hct, Hgb, blood chemistries and electrolytes sent to lab stat, and abdominal films obtained.
Results pending.

Patient to be transferred from gastroenterology clinic to unit via wheelchair with RN in attendance."

Figure 9.3	*Pediatric unit teachable moments (cont.)*

Case 3

Who-When-What-Think-Ask-Do

Who, what, when: The new schedule in the pulmonary clinic has just been posted for next month, and the nurse sees that he or she is scheduled to perform follow-up phone calls and home visits for patients discharged from the hospital during the past month. Some home visits are in neighborhoods with high crime rates.

Think: The nurse is able to identify the outcome criteria for the various home visits:

- Physiologic recovery of the patient
- Understanding of home management and adherence to treatment regimen
- Effective patient/family adjustment

Ask: The nurse should ask how to prioritize care. Is he or she competent in performing all procedures, assessments, physical care counseling, and guidance that may be necessary during the home visit or should he or she seek out a mentor/preceptor to assist with skill-building in advance of the assignment?

Do: The nurse **reviews** the discharge summary, lab values, physician orders, and the teaching plan noting any special needs of the child/teen/family, or any unique family dynamic prior to the home visit.

The nurse **collects** all necessary equipment, teaching materials, and supplies, and ensures they are clean, adequate for the intended purpose, and in working order.

The nurse **obtains** directions to the families' homes and, if necessary, performs a trial run before the appointed visit in order to be on time.

 ©2007 HCPro, Inc.   **Critical Thinking in the Pediatric Unit**

Figure

9.3

Pediatric unit teachable moments (cont.)

The nurse **provides** for personal safety by giving the hospital a copy of the full daily itinerary before leaving for the home visit.

The nurse **reports** to the hospital at intervals during the day and may choose to visit with another team member in especially dangerous areas.

The nurse will use **common sense** in guiding his or her actions in dangerous areas. If intuition says a place/situation is unsafe the nurse will leave immediately and report the situation to authorities.

Case 4

Who-When-What-Think-Ask-Do

Who, what, when: A 10-month-old male is admitted with a femur fracture following a motor vehicle crash. He is asleep when the orthopedic surgeon comes in to see him on rounds. Shortly after the surgeon leaves the room, the child wakes up crying and cannot be consoled despite having received medication for pain two hours ago.

The patient's hospital course has been uneventful and the fracture is healing nicely.

The patient's mother comes out to the nurses' station and demands that her child be given something else for pain.

The nurse contacts the surgeon on call who refuses to write additional orders for pain medication for the patient.

Think: The nurse recognizes that the orders for this patient's pain management are not effectively managing the child's pain. The nurse knows that the provider can be unapproachable at times and even overtly demeaning to nurses. The nurse knows that a possible/probable confrontation can be avoided by following the orders given, yet also knows that the first priority is the comfort of the child and the best interest of the patient and family.

Figure 9.3	*Pediatric unit teachable moments (cont.)*

The nurse considers intervening on the patient's behalf and offering the provider other "suggestions" for this patient:

- Coming to reevaluate the patient during the painful episode
- Increasing the dose or frequency of the medication ordered
- Changing to another medication that will more effectively manage the child's pain
- Requesting that the Pain Management Service be consulted

Ask: What course of action should the nurse take?

Do: Collaboratively approach provider with "suggestions."

- Develop a plan of care for this patient to make the pain assessment, intervention, and reassessment cycle a priority
- Trying some non-pharmacologic interventions to assist in managing the child's pain
- Continue to communicate ineffective pain control to the provider. If no change in response, escalate communication up the chain of command

Source: June Marshall, RN, MS, CNAA,BC

Figure

9.4

Pediatric case studies

Pediatric case studies displaying critical thinking

Critical thinking in the emergency department

A 17-year-old female, a patient of the pediatric clinic, arrives ambulatory in the emergency department accompanied by a male companion. Her chief complaint is, "My stomach is killing me and is as hard as a rock." The patient is taken by herself to the exam room.

Inquisitive

Asks questions:

- When did the pain start?
- What were you doing when it started?
- How long has your stomach been hard?
- When was your last menstrual period?
- When was the last time you 'partied?'
- Have you been physically, verbally, or emotionally abused or injured by anyone?
- When did you last have sexual relations of any kind?
- Is there anything you think that I should know or that you want to tell me?

If the patient is not a drug user/abuser it's better that the patient suffer the indignity of questions related to drug use than miss the opportunity of putting a drug user/abuser at ease by asking open-ended questions that he or she is less apt to answer honestly.

Self-confident

Initiates action by:

- Notifying the ED physician to see the patient
- Notifying the Social Worker to see the patient and contact the parents
- Completing a pregnancy test according to hospital protocol before sending the patient to radiology

Gathers supplies to complete lab draws and start IV in anticipation of physician orders

Figure	
9.4	*Pediatric case studies (cont.)*

Analytical

Uses reason and logic:

- Observes dilated pupils, headache, blurred vision, abdominal pain, increase in vital signs, and is able to palpate a rigid abdomen. Suspects these signs indicate possible cocaine use

Systematic

Organized, a fixed approach to problem solving:

- Observes and assesses while at the same time moves forward taking action

Open-minded

Accepting and non-judgmental:

- Ensures all possible comfort of the patient by acceptance of her possible diversity of lifestyle

Truth seeking

Asks any question comfortably:

- Asks about possible drug use, sexual relations, and the possibility of abuse both openly and comfortably

Critical thinking during pediatric patient transport

You are transporting a 2-year-old critically ill patient in respiratory distress, via ambulance, from a small community hospital to a tertiary care pediatric center in the city. The ambulance has come upon a complete traffic back-up on the expressway and the patient starts to deteriorate.

Inquisitive

Asks questions:

- What's the status of the traffic jam?
- Can the ambulance driver radio for information on the traffic problem?
- Does the patient exhibit any signs that he may require intubation?
- Is there a way around the traffic jam, legal or otherwise?

Figure	*Pediatric case studies (cont.)*
9.4	

Systematic

Organized, a fixed approach to problem solving:

- Considered the child's status
- Collects data on traffic jam
- Prepares alternative plan for moving forward in a timely manner

Analytical

Uses reason and logic:

- Is the child's airway stable enough to make it to the facility without the child arresting?
- If the patient arrests in the ambulance, what should the nurse do to ensure safe passage to the pediatric center for the child?

Self-confident

Initiates action by:

The pediatric nurse tells the ambulance driver to pull over to the shoulder of the expressway, turn on the lights but no siren, drive on the shoulder and pass the traffic back-up, pull off at the next off-ramp and take city streets to the tertiary care center using both lights and siren.

Critical thinking on the pediatric unit

J.S. is a 14-year-old admitted yesterday for a perforated appendix. J.S. is a student at a middle school in the next county and lives with her mother and father. At report you were told that J.S. refuses to get out of bed and is crying despite receiving therapeutic opioid doses. Her father has been at her side since admission and provided support for her. Her mother has not been in to see her. When you enter the room to complete the assessment, you find the father lying in bed with her. The surgeon who performed the appendectomy has asked for a gynecology consult, because he visualized inflamed fallopian tubes at the time of surgery and is concerned that the patient also has pelvic inflammatory disease.

Figure 9.4	Pediatric case studies (cont.)

Inquisitive

Asks questions:

- Why can't or won't the patient get out of bed?
- Why isn't the opioid being given providing adequate pain control?
- Is there any sign of abdominal infection, either active or impending?
- What was the blood loss during the procedure?
- Why hasn't the patient's mother been to see her?
- Why didn't the patient's father provide her with privacy during the gynecologist's exam?

Systematic

Organized, a fixed approach to problem solving:

- Reads the operative report for estimated blood loss
- Checks lab results on the chart for results of today's CBC
- Asks patient's father to leave the room while postoperative assessment is performed
- Observes father's demeanor when asked to leave the room
- Notices that patient remains facing the wall and avoids interaction of any kind
- Forms a rapport with the patient while performing assessment
- Observes that patient exhibits extreme modesty and cries easily while holding blanket up to her neck
- Informs patient that you will be assisting her to get out of bed shortly and ask if she requires any pain medication beforehand

Truth seeking

- Asks any question comfortably
- Asks the patient why she doesn't want to get out of bed
- Asks the patient if she knows why her mother has not visited her
- Asks the patient is she has ever had sexual relations
- Asks the patient if she has ever used birth control
- Asks the patient if her mother will be in to visit
- Asks the patient about her relationship with her father

Figure	*Pediatric case studies (cont.)*
9.4	

Analytical

Uses reason and logic:

- Patient seems very immature for a 14-year-old
- Patient doesn't want to look anyone in the eyes
- Patient is overly modest, even for a teenager
- Patient refuses to get out of bed or take part in any of her own care
- The patient's father is very reluctant to leave the room while the nurse is caring for the patient
- Patient's mother refuses to visit the patient
- The surgeon is concerned the patient has pelvic inflammatory disease

Self-confident

Initiates action by:

Based on the data collection, the patient's behavior, the father's reluctance to leave the patient's side at any time, the patient's mother's refusal to visit, the patient's heightened modesty and apparent estrangement from her mother, the nurse requests a consult with the physician, the social services team, and the hospital psychologist to rule out the possibility of incest.

Critical thinking in the NICU

You are a new pool nurse in a children's hospital with a neonatal intensive care unit (NICU). Today you are assigned to the NICU due to an increase in the census and a shortage of NICU nurses due to illness. You have recently completed your required neonatal advanced life support (NALS) course and are currently taking the required neonatal courses that are included in pediatric orientation. The charge nurse assigns a 32-week neonate with necrotizing enterocolitis who is on a ventilator to your care.

Inquisitive

Asks questions:

- What is entailed in taking care of this patient?
- Will I be taking care of this patient alone or may I share this assignment with a permanent member of the NICU staff?
- Do I know what I don't know?

Critical Thinking in the Pediatric Unit

©2007 HCPro, Inc.

Figure

9.4

Pediatric case studies (cont.)

- How do I feel about taking this assignment?
- Will someone be available if phlebotomy needs to be performed on this patient or if new IV access needs to be obtained?

Systematic

Organized, a fixed approach to problem solving:

- Mentally review what I know, and don't know about NEC and the pulmonary system of a 32-week preemie
- Receive report from night shift
- Ask questions about the report given
- Make walking rounds with the night shift nurse
- Check the patient and all tubes, lines, and equipment
- Verify well-being and patency of IV access
- Check the chart for new orders that may not have been noted

Truth seeking

Asks any question comfortably:

- Ask yourself: Am I qualified to take this assignment?
- Discuss the assignment with the charge nurse
- Let the charge nurse know of your apprehension so that he or she can support your needs and decisions

Analytical

Uses reason and logic:

- I have been given the information about NEC and ventilators in my neonatal courses
- Although I am a pool nurse I've chosen to take the pediatric track, which includes assignments to the NICU
- The hospital has provided me with the necessary courses to ensure my competency
- I have taken full advantage of these learning opportunities
- Support will be given if I should need it

 ©2007 HCPro, Inc.

Figure	*Pediatric case studies (cont.)*
9.4	

Self-confident

Initiates action by:

- I feel competent that I can transfer the learning into practice safely
- I feel comfortable with the support provided by the charge nurse
- I feel that this will be my initiation into NICU nursing

Critical thinking in the pediatric clinic

C.G. is a 9-year-old female patient of the pediatric clinic. She is obese and has a diagnosis of Type 2 diabetes. Her parents both work outside the home, and her 75-year-old grandmother stays with her after school. Her daily diet is high in fat and complex carbohydrates, and her snacks consist of chips and candy. She is at the clinic today with her parents to meet with a registered dietitian for help in making better choices in her daily diet. C.G. and her family live in a mobile home with eight other relatives. Their home is located an hour from the city. C.G. is often wearing torn clothing that is too small for her and she exhibits poor hygiene. C.G.'s father works in construction and her mother cleans houses for a living.

When you enter the room to greet C.G., you find her teary eyed and distraught. Her parents are quietly speaking to each other in Spanish. You sit down next to her and give her a hug. When she is able to stop crying she refuses to talk, though she speaks English proficiently.

The Spanish-speaking dietitian arrives and begins diet counseling with C.G. and her parents. At the end of the session the dietitian comes to you and tells you that she noticed lice in C.G.'s hair. C.G. is now weeping uncontrollably. What actions should you take?

Inquisitive

Asks questions:

- When did C.G. eat last and what is her blood sugar?
- Were C.G. and her parents receptive to the dietitian's teaching?
- What exactly did the dietitian see in C.G.'s hair?
- Is she sure that what she saw are actually lice?

<table>
<tr><td>Figure
9.4</td><td>Pediatric case studies (cont.)</td></tr>
</table>

- Did she tell C.G. and her parents what she saw?

- Why is C.G. crying? Is it about the lice, about her dietary restrictions, or about something else?

- Do I now harbor lice in MY hair?

Systematic

Organized, a fixed approach to problem solving:

- Identify and prioritize C.G.'s problems:

  1. Poor diet control

  2. Unsanitary living conditions

  3. Possible head lice

- Assess C.G.'s head for lice and ask the pediatrician to confirm

Truth seeking

Asks any question comfortably:

- Ask C.G. why she is crying

- Ask C.G. if she remembers any one thing the dietitian told her about her food choices

- Ask C.G. if she has noticed anything in her hair or if other kids at school or at home have had head lice

- Ask C.G. if she knows what head lice look like

- Ask C.G. if she has ever had head lice

Analytical

Uses reason and logic:

- C.G. probably did not retain the dietitian's teaching because she was upset

- C.G.'s parents may not support the dietary restrictions

- C.G.'s nutritional counseling needs to be rescheduled ASAP

- It is very probable that what the dietitian saw in C.G.'s hair are lice

- It is possible that the nurse may have acquired head lice while consoling C.G.

Figure 9.4	*Pediatric case studies (cont.)*

Self-confident

Initiates action by:

- Having C.G. remain in the exam room
- Having C.G.'s mom check C.G.'s blood sugar
- Rescheduling C.G.'s diet teaching
- Calling social services for assistance in obtaining school and community resources for C.G. and her family
- Notifying the medical provider to examine the parents for lice and obtain an order for pediculicidal shampoo for C.G. and her family to use
- Allowing C.G. to use the showers in the hospital to shampoo and provide her with a scrub suit to wear until her own clothing can be obtained and washed appropriately
- Encouraging the parents to have all other family members living in the home examined for lice
- Providing instructions for the family regarding disinfecting the home and treating other family members
- Calling housekeeping for disinfection of the exam room after C.G. leaves
- Obtaining an appropriate pediculicidal shampoo from the hospital pharmacy for the nurse and change scrubs before leaving the hospital

Source: June Marshall, RN, MS, CNAA,BC

Figure **9.5**	*Sample agenda*

[Your facility] Critical Thinking Skills
[Date of program]

9:00–9:15	Introduction to critical thinking and course overview
9:15–10:00	Patient assessments
	Anatomy/physiology review
	Establishing the baseline
	Reassessments
10:00–10:15	Stretch break
10:15–11:30	Age-specific patients
	Include pediatric and/or geriatric specifics
	Geriatric
	Polypharmacy issues
	Atypical presentations
	Elder misuse and reporting
	Pediatric
	Social challenges
	Children as victims and reporting suspicion
	Medication specifics for children
11:30–12:15	Lunch
12:15–1:15	Red flags
	Patient statements/comments
	Family input
	Documentation specifics
	Case scenarios
1:15–1:30	Stretch break
1:30–2:30	Applying the knowledge
	When to call the doctor
	More case scenarios
2:30	Course evaluations

Source: Shelley Cohen, RN, BS, CEN

Figure 9.6	**Instructor worksheet—Connecting words to spark critical thinking**

In each of these patient cases, what question(s) should you consider?

(Instructor notes: What to ask or what you want the nurse to consider.)

1. Child continues to cry after the medication you gave him for pain.

   (Instructor note: Why is there no pain relief?)

2. Six month old infant has poor weight gain. Mother states she feeds the child frequently, but he is a poor eater.

   (Instructor note: Any other signs and symptoms of note? What questions should you ask the parent? What evaluations can be done to collect further data?)

3. Patient is having large amounts of drainage on the abdominal dressing.

   (Instructor note: How frequently is the dressing being changed? Is each nurse assessing by the same standard as provided in the hospital policy and procedure for quantifying wound drainage?)

4. Child is having difficulty breathing.

   (Instructor note: What physical signs and symptoms must be assessed? What non-invasive procedures can evaluate effectiveness of respirations?)

Source: Shelley Cohen, RN, BS, CEN and June Marshall, RN, MS, CNAA,BC

Figure 9.7	Nurse worksheet—Connecting words to spark critical thinking

Following each of these patient statements, what question(s) should you consider?

1. Patient's mother states that he is still crying and has had no pain relief after the medication you gave him or her.

2. Six-month-old infant has poor weight gain. Mother states she feeds the child frequently but he is a poor eater.

3. Patient is having large amounts of drainage on the abdominal dressing following intestinal surgery.

4. Mother states the child is struggling harder to breathe today.

Source: Shelley Cohen, RN, BS, CEN and June Marshall, RN, MS, CNAA,BC

Figure 9.8	*Worksheet—Relationship to critical thinking*

How does each of these items below relate to critical thinking? Give one patient example for each.

Invasive and non-invasive therapy/treatment/indwelling devices

- Intravenous access devices and therapy
  - peripheral IV catheters
  - PICC lines
  - fluids/parenteral nutrition
  - blood products

- Catheters
  - Foley
  - In and out catheterization

- Feeding tubes
  - Nasogastric
  - Gastrostomy

- Surgical dressings and wound drains

- Physiologic monitoring
  - cardiac/apnea monitor
  - pulse oximetry

- Pain management
  - patient controlled analgesia
  - non-pharmacologic pain management

- Respiratory therapy
  - aerosolized medications
  - oxygen therapy

Source: Shelley Cohen, RN, BS, CEN and June Marshall, RN, MS, CNAA,BC

Figure
9.9

Worksheet—Vital signs

In each set of pediatric vital signs below, what question would you ask the patient/parent? What other areas would you assess?

Vital signs + Assessment = Critical thinking

"A critical thinker is able to reject information that is incorrect or irrelevant." —S. Ferrett

Case 1: 1 month old

Temp	96.2°F
Pulse	124
Respirations	30
Blood pressure	96/68

Case 2: 3 year old

Temp	101.9°F
Pulse	100
Respirations	24
Blood pressure	116/76

Case 3: 12 year old

Temp	100.4°F
Pulse	92
Respirations	28
Blood pressure	130/88

Source: Shelley Cohen, RN, BS, CEN and June Marshall, RN, MS, CNAA,BC

Figure **9.10**	***Worksheet—Red flag alerts***

Patient statement/question	Makes you think . . .	Your response is . . .
My baby feels really hot and vomits everything I feed her.		
My boyfriend gets very angry every time my son wets the bed.		
My child is really irritable and keeps pulling at his ears.		
My baby got this bruise when he fell off the sofa.		
My little girl says it hurts when she goes to the bathroom.		
My stomach hurts a lot, and I want my mom to come get me at school and take me home.		
My teenage daughter keeps losing weight, and I don't know what to do.		
Please help me. My baby is having trouble breathing.		

Source: Shelley Cohen, RN, BS, CEN and June Marshall, RN, MS, CNAA,BC

Figure
9.11

Worksheet—Relating nursing care to critical thinking

For each of the following skills, procedures, or interventions, answer the questions below:

- IV access/therapy
- Cardiac/respiratory monitoring
- Enteral feeding via nasogastric tube
- Nasopharyngeal/oropharyngeal suctioning
- Pain assessment and management
- Medical immobilization (use of restraints)
- Obtaining blood and urine specimens in infants or young children
- Taking a sexual history in a late school aged child or adolescent
- Reporting suspected abuse or neglect

1. Why would the patient need this?

2. What is my role in this?

3. How will I know it's safe?

4. Will I be able to adequately assess the efficacy of this procedure/intervention?

5. What are the risks/benefits of this?

6. What observations/considerations should I make in regard to this intervention?

7. Does the patient have any cultural/ethnic beliefs or practices that will have an effect on this procedure/intervention?

8. Will this procedure/intervention impact negatively on the intra/interfamily privacy issues?

Source: Marie Lawless-Shipley, RN, BC; MSN, CNS and June Marshall, RN, MS, CNAA,BC

Figure	*Pediatric nurses and critical thinking*
9.12	

Pediatric nurses demonstrate critical thinking by doing the following:

- Looking for signs of abnormal growth and development
- Asking each parent safety questions at each visit to identify concerns regarding the child's home environment
- Identifying issues and concerns regarding parent-child relationships
- Recognizing signs and symptoms of physiologic and psychologic distress
- Preparing and teaching parenting classes
- Identifying and reporting signs and symptoms of physical, emotional, and/or sexual abuse
- Researching a new procedure and writing an evidence-based protocol for implementation
- Applying knowledge of anatomy, physiology, microbiology, genetics, and immunology when assessing a patient
- Anticipating the patient/family needs based upon assessment findings
- Making referrals to other team members such as child life specialists, social workers, school personnel, and chaplains to assist in addressing identified needs
- Delegating aspects of care to unlicensed assistive personnel
- Assessing and managing pain
- Creating and maintaining a safe environment to prevent risk of injury
- Conveying information concisely, accurately, and efficiently
- Evaluating effectiveness of interventions
- Providing just-in-time parent education from the time of admission through discharge

Source: Marie Lawless-Shipley, RN, BC; MSN, CNS and June Marshall, RN, MS, CNAA, BC

Nursing education instructional guide

Target audience

- Chief nursing officers
- Directors of nursing
- Nurse managers
- Directors of education
- Staff development specialists
- VPs of nursing
- Nurse preceptors
- HR professionals

Statement of need

This practical guide to teaching and developing critical thinking includes strategies for designing and holding critical thinking courses, how to include critical thinking training in orientation, and how to encourage the ongoing development of critical thinking. Critical thinking skills help nurses become better decision makers and encourage independent practice. The book teaches nurse leaders, nurse managers, and staff educators how to develop critical thinking in the classroom and on the unit so they can incorporate critical thinking into everyday practice, both for novice nurses and ongoing development for advanced practitioners. (This activity is intended for individual use only.)

Educational objectives

Upon completion of this activity, participants should be able to

- Describe the characteristics of the pediatric unit that require good critical-thinking skills
- Identify key aspects of critical thinking
- Explain how nurses develop competency in critical thinking
- Analyze the factors that contribute to new graduates' lack of critical thinking
- Identify strategies to facilitate critical thinking in new graduates
- Determine classroom strategies to teach, promote, and support the development of critical thinking
- Determine ways to evaluate nurses' progress in critical thinking throughout orientation
- Develop strategies for the development of critical thinking skills during the orientation process
- Discuss the role played by managers and educators in promoting environments that support critical thinking
- Analyze the challenges that both new and experienced nurses face in the incorporation of critical thinking skills in the practice setting
- Explain interventions to help both new and experienced nurses meet their managers and preceptors expectations for critical thinking
- Apply critical thinking to nursing documentation

Faculty

Shelley Cohen, RN, BS, CEN, is the founder and president of Health Resources Unlimited, a Tennessee-based healthcare education and consulting company *(www.hru.net)*. Through her seminars for nursing professionals, Cohen coaches and educates healthcare workers and leaders across the country to provide the very best in patient care. She frequently presents her work on leadership and triage at national conferences.

She has a background in emergency, critical care, and occupational medicine. Over the past 30 years, she has worked both as a staff nurse and nurse executive.

 ©2007 HCPro, Inc. **Critical Thinking in the Pediatric Unit**

Polly Gerber Zimmermann, RN, MS, MBA, CEN, has been in active in emergency and medical-surgical nursing clinical practice for more than 29 years and involved in nurse educating for more than 10 years. She was the senior course manager for the nursing division of the National Center for Advanced Medical Education, and is a tenured assistant professor in the Department of Nursing at the Harry S. Truman College (Chicago). Under her guidance, the school's curriculum instituted an integration of prioritization principles and critical thinking that resulted in the school's students improving from below to above national average results in these areas on standardized test scores.

June Marshall, RN, MS, CNAA,BC has been a pediatric nurse for more than 33 years, and has worked in a variety of roles including staff nurse, clinical nurse specialist, adjunct faculty, entrepreneur, and nurse administrator. She has worked in inpatient, ambulatory, rehabilitation, and home care settings. She has also lectured and served as a preceptor for undergraduate and graduate students in pediatric nursing in a variety of clinical settings.

Accreditation/designation statement

This educational activity for three nursing contact hours is provided by HCPro, Inc. HCPro is accredited as a provider of continuing nursing education by the American Nurses Credentialing Center Commission on Accreditation.

Disclosure statements

HCPro, Inc. has a conflict-of-interest policy that requires course faculty to disclose any real or apparent commercial financial affiliations related to the content of their presentations/materials. It is not assumed that these financial interests or affiliations will have an adverse impact on faculty presentations; they are simply noted here to fully inform the participants.

Shelley Cohen, Polly Gerber Zimmermann, and June Marshall have declared that they have no commercial/ financial vested interest in this activity.

Instructions

In order to be eligible to receive your nursing contact hours for this activity, you are required to do the following:

1. Read the book *Critical Thinking in the Pediatric Unit: Skills to Assess, Analyze, and Act*
2. Complete the exam
3. Complete the evaluation
4. Provide your contact information on the exam and evaluation
5. Submit exam and evaluation to HCPro, Inc.

Please provide all of the information requested above and mail or fax your completed exam, program evaluation, and contact information to

HCPro, Inc.
Attention: Continuing Education Department
200 Hoods Lane
P.O. Box 1168
Marblehead, MA 01945
Fax: 781/639-0179

NOTE:

This book and associated exam are intended for individual use only. If you would like to provide this continuing education exam to other members of your nursing staff, please contact our customer service department at 877/727-1728 to place your order. The exam fee schedule is as follows:

Exam quantity	Fee
1	$ 0
2–25	$15 per person
26–50	$12 per person
51–100	$ 8 per person
101+	$ 5 per person

Continuing education exam

Name: _____

Title: _____

Facility name: _____

Address: _____

Address: _____

City: _____ State: _____ Zip: _____

Phone number: _____ Fax number: _____

E-mail: _____

Nursing license number: _____

(ANCC requires a unique identifier for each learner.)

Date completed: _____

1. **When floating to an unfamiliar unit, nurses in pediatric settings must function in**

    a. narrowly-defined roles, caring for a specific age group of children

    b. cross-trained roles as part of a multidisciplinary team

    c. isolation to other departments

    d. accordance with guidelines recommended by the healthcare facility

2. **The most successful pediatric nurses are those who**

    a. are analytical and able to respect the values and cultures of others

    b. are technically competent and single-minded

    c. have many years of experience in nursing

    d. have strong beliefs about the best way to parent children

3. **When nurses are working in pediatrics, it is most important they possess which of the following skills?**

    a. Basic knowledge in growth and development

    b. Strong delegation skills

    c. Good telephone communication skills

    d. The ability to make good clinical decisions based on sound professional judgment

4. **According to Benner, a nurse that views a situation as a whole rather than in parts and is able to develop a solution is:**

    a. advanced beginner

    b. competent

    c. proficient

    d. technical

5. **According to Del Bueno's definition of critical thinking, which of the following is an essential aspect in a clinical setting?**

    a. The nurse thinks outside the box to create a novel nursing approach

    b. The nurse can state the five rights of all types of medication administration

    c. The nurse can define the meaning of ABCD prioritization

    d. The nurse does the right thing for the right reason

6. **A new graduate nurse that has little confidence in his or her skills and decision-making abilities has**

    a. unfamiliarity with the structure of the organization

    b. lack of clinical judgment

    c. lack of professional relationships

    d. lack of professional training

7. **To minimize the stress of new graduate nurses, consider**

    a. handing out stress balls during orientation

    b. suggesting they wait, assess, and hope for a solution

    c. using a mentor or assigning a buddy who builds a relationship and follows the nurse for at least one year

    d. avoiding support groups that introduce graduate nurses to the worries and stresses of their peers

8. **True sudden beginning of symptoms can signal a catastrophic event. Which prioritization principle can this be applied to?**

    a. Trends

    b. Systemic over local

    c. Actual over potential

    d. Onset

9. **To help new graduates identify worst-case scenarios,**

    a. give examples of actual cases and identify the worst-case complications

    b. have the new graduates witness worst-case scenarios

    c. discuss ethical consequences if worst-case scenarios are missed

    d. teach basic pathophysiology

10. **Aids to help create a classroom-learning environment include:**

    a. use of a podium during presentations to communicate an air of expert authority

    b. avoiding the use of color as it distracts the learner from paying attention to the speaker

    c. having a break every 90-120 minutes to avoid breaking the learners' concentration

    d. placement of posters around the classroom walls to promote learning even if the learners' eyes wander

11. **Which of the following would be most likely to help motivate a Generation X nurse learn?**

    a. Relate the material to a sense of duty to keep current

    b. Emphasize the role of authority of the expert instructor

    c. Play games as a method to teach the material

    d. Focus on the possibility of future promotions if learning is evident

12. **When new graduates are asked about their biggest fears and concerns about becoming professional nurses, they frequently mention**

    a. how to communicate with physicians

    b. they will be late for work

    c. they will feel left out and have trouble making friends at work

    d. they can't safely administer meds

13. Unfolding case scenarios provide information in staggered amounts, followed by

    a. outcomes

    b. results

    c. answers

    d. questions

14. In cooperative learning, the advantage of a "think, pair, and share" exercise is that everyone

    a. participates

    b. has an opinion

    c. memorizes the objective

    d. develops a relationship

15. Which of the following is an effective way to use questions in a classroom setting?

    a. Ask trick questions

    b. Pose questions to stimulate thinking rather than yes/no questions

    c. Always let the most outspoken student answer

    d. Limit all questions to the end of class

16. When developing a self-assessment tool for new graduate nurses to measure their perception of their ability to perform at the critical thinking level, it is best to include items that reflect

    a. recall of information

    b. personality traits

    c. generic nursing skill

    d. history of the institution

17. As new nurses work through the orientation process, evaluating their ability to apply critical thinking in their clinical setting needs to be

    a. evidenced

    b. difficult

    c. strict

    d. general

18. **Preceptors can help orientees develop and stimulate the use of critical thinking skills by**

    a. minimizing emphasis on the ability to recognize when the skill or talk is needed

    b. discouraging realistic time frames

    c. assuming the new hire understands the what, why, how, and when of delivering nursing care

    d. minimizing the emphasis on ability to perform skills and tasks

19. **When nursing staff other than the preceptor are working with the orientee, it is _____ that the preceptor educates all staff on the importance of their role in assisting with the transition process of the newly hired nurse.**

    a. not important

    b. essential

    c. somewhat important

    d. unnecessary

20. **Managers and educators need to ensure a patient care environment that nurtures critical thinkers, stimulates them, and motivates them to engage in a discussion in their minds. This discussion is all about which of the following questions?**

    a. Is this in the best interest of the organization?

    b. Is this in the best interest of myself?

    c. Is this in the best interest of the patient?

    d. Is this in the best interest of my learning process?

21. **When considering how to improve the content of job descriptions, nurse managers should ask staff**

    a. what they do on a regular basis that is not part of the job description

    b. to write a list of their favorite tasks

    c. to edit the job description

    d. nothing—nurse managers should not ask staff for assistance in improving the content of job descriptions

22. A challenge that new graduate nurses face upon entering the workplace that directly affects their critical thinking abilities is

    a. students have had too much clinical experience in school

    b. many nurses today enter a specialty straight out of school, rather than gaining years of experience first

    c. students have had so much clinical time that they have been exposed to too many challenging patients

    d. students today do not have to contend with a shortage of nursing faculty

23. To coach new graduate nurses through bad patient outcomes

    a. do not allow them to have any grieving time through their error/omission

    b. even if the bad outcome was not related to something they did or did not do, allow a guilt trip to help them cope

    c. allow others to debrief the nurses before you do

    d. provide them with more than one opportunity to sit with a supportive mentor or preceptor to review the scenario that led to the patient outcome

24. To encourage collaborative efforts between the medical staff and new graduate nurses

    a. avoid introducing new graduates to too many members of the medical staff to avoid overwhelming the new graduates

    b. do not allow medical staff that has had previous negative experiences with new graduate nurses to interact with the new graduate nurses.

    c. ask the medical staff to think back to their own internships and remind them that new graduate's critical thinking will develop with their support

    d. have new graduates in specialty areas stay out of practitioner offices

25. Transforming critical thinking into the written format provides a legal record to support nurse's

    a. patient outcomes related to any intervention

    b. right to work

    c. attendance

    d. ability to follow directions

Continuing education evaluation

Name: _____

Title: _____

Facility name: _____

Address: _____

Address:_____

City: _____ **State:** _____ **Zip:** _____

Phone number: _____ **Fax number:** _____

E-mail: _____

Nursing license number: _____

(ANCC requires a unique identifier for each learner.)

Date completed: _____

1. **This activity met the learning objectives stated:**

   Strongly agree   Agree   Disagree   Strongly disagree

2. **Objectives were related to the overall purpose/goal of the activity:**

   Strongly agree   Agree   Disagree   Strongly disagree

3. **This activity was related to my continuing education needs:**

   Strongly agree   Agree   Disagree   Strongly disagree

4. **The exam for the activity was an accurate test of the knowledge gained:**

   Strongly agree   Agree   Disagree   Strongly disagree

5. **The activity avoided commercial bias or influence:**

   Strongly agree   Agree   Disagree   Strongly disagree

6. **This activity met my expectations:**

       Strongly agree   Agree   Disagree   Strongly disagree

7. **Will this activity enhance your professional practice?**

       Yes   No

8. **The format was an appropriate method for delivery of the content for this activity:**

       Strongly agree   Agree   Disagree   Strongly disagree

9. **If you have any comments on this activity, please note them here:**

10. **How much time did it take for you to complete this activity?**

Thank you for completing this evaluation of our continuing education activity!

Return completed form to:

HCPro, Inc. • Attention: Continuing Education Department • 200 Hoods Lane, Marblehead, MA 01945
Telephone: 877/727-1728 • Fax: 781/639-2982